DOWN SYNDROME WITH LOVE

A PRACTICAL GUIDE TO UPBRINGING

DR. A. MITRA MBBS, MD, DMI

Disclaimer:

The information provided in this book is intended for educational purposes only. While every effort has been made to ensure accuracy and relevance, readers are advised to consult healthcare professionals for personalized advice and treatment options tailored to individual circumstances. The author and publisher disclaim any liability arising directly or indirectly from the use or application of the contents of this book.

ISBN:

DEDICATION

To the incredible individuals with Down syndrome who inspire us every day, and to the devoted parents and caregivers who love and support them unconditionally. This book is for you. May it be a source of knowledge, comfort, and joy on your remarkable journey together.

CONTENTS

ACKNOWLEDGMENTS

My deepest appreciation goes to the parents, educators, therapists, and medical professionals who form the unwavering support system for individuals with Down syndrome. Your expertise and compassion are an inspiration. A heartfelt thank you to the families who shared their experiences, your openness enriches this book and will undoubtedly guide others on their path. Finally, to my own source of love and support, thank you for believing in this project.

1. WELCOMING YOUR SUPER SPECIAL CHILD

Embracing the Journey with Love

Finding out your precious child has Down syndrome can feel like the ground has shifted beneath your feet. A whirlwind of emotions might take hold – confusion, fear, sadness, a million questions swirling in your mind. "What does this mean for my child? What will their life be like?" This chapter is here to offer a warm embrace and guide you through this initial wave.

A Unique Spectrum of Abilities

Down syndrome occurs when a person has an extra copy of chromosome 21. This genetic difference can cause some physical and developmental differences, but it is important to remember that it does not define your child. Every child experiences Down syndrome in their own unique way.

Here are some things you might see:

- **Distinctive Features:** Some common physical characteristics associated with Down syndrome include a round face, slanted eyes with folds at the inner corners (epicanthal folds), a small nose, and a single line across the palm of the hand (simian crease). However, these features can vary considerably.

- **Developmental Differences:** Some children with Down syndrome might have learning delays that need extra support. They might learn to roll over, crawl, walk, or talk a little later than other children. They might also have trouble with things like balance, coordination, or speech.

- **Strengths and Talents:** It is crucial to remember that Down syndrome is a spectrum. While some children might face challenges, others might excel in specific areas like music, art, memory, or social interaction. Every child has their own unique set of strengths and talents waiting to be discovered.

The Diagnosis: A New Chapter, Not an Ending

A diagnosis might feel daunting, but it is a starting point, not an ending. Now you have the knowledge to access a wealth of resources designed to help your child thrive.

- **Early Intervention:** Starting early is key! Early intervention programs can provide therapies like physical, occupational, and speech therapy. These therapies can help your child develop important skills like communication, movement, and social interaction.

- **Support Groups:** Connecting with other families who have children with Down syndrome is invaluable. You can share experiences, learn from each other, and build a strong support network.

- **Educators and Therapists:** Your pediatrician, therapists, and child's educators will become your partners in this journey. They will provide guidance and support to help you create an individualized plan for your child's development.

Focusing on Your Child's Strengths

Instead of dwelling on the challenges, let us celebrate all the amazing things about your child! Perhaps they have a radiant smile that melts hearts, a laugh that is contagious and fills the room with joy, or a remarkable ability to focus intently on a toy or activity. These are their strengths – let them shine! As you celebrate your child's unique abilities, you will discover a world of wonder and unconditional love in your relationship.

Building Your Support System

The path ahead may feel like a winding road at times,

but remember, you do not have to walk it alone. Here are some ways to build a strong support system:

- **Connect with Families:** Seek out families who have children with Down syndrome. You can find them online, through support groups, or through recommendations from your doctor. Sharing experiences and knowledge can be incredibly helpful.

- **Talk to Your Doctor:** Your pediatrician is a vital resource. Ask questions, express your concerns, and work together to create a care plan that addresses your child's specific needs.

- **Involve Educators and Therapists:** Your child's teachers and therapists are dedicated to your child's success. Build strong relationships with them, communicate openly, and work collaboratively to create an inclusive learning environment.

Love is the Foundation

Above all else, remember the incredible power of love. Your child thrives on affection, acceptance, and a safe and nurturing environment. Here are some ways to shower them with love:

- **Create a Loving Routine:** Establish routines that provide comfort and predictability. This can include things like bedtime stories, cuddles, and playtime.

- **Celebrate Every Milestone:** Every accomplishment, big or small, is a reason to celebrate! This will boost your child's confidence and motivate them to learn and grow.

- **Positive Reinforcement:** Focus on positive reinforcement. When your child tries their best or achieves a goal, celebrate it! This will encourage them to keep trying and reach their full potential.

- **Unconditional Love:** Let your child know you love them unconditionally, no matter what. This will provide them with a strong foundation of security and self-worth.

This chapter is just the beginning of your incredible journey. It is a call to celebrate your unique child, build a strong support network.

2. COMMUNICATION, DEVELOPMENT, AND SELF-ESTEEM

Your child with Down syndrome is a blossoming superstar! This chapter dives deep into the essential building blocks that will empower them to reach their full potential: communication, development, and self-esteem. We'll explore practical strategies and celebrate the unique ways your child learns and grows.

Communication

Communication is a beautiful dance of expressing ourselves and understanding others. Here are some ways to help your child become a confident communicator:

- **Tailoring Your Communication Style:** Every child learns differently. Pay attention to your child's cues. If they respond well to visuals, incorporate picture cards, sign language, or photos into your conversations. Short, clear sentences with repetition will be easier for them to understand.

- **The Power of Play:** Playtime is not just fun; it is a communication powerhouse! Engage your child in pretend play, where they can practice social interaction and communication skills. Sing songs, tell stories with different voices, and create interactive games that encourage turn-taking and listening.

- **Interactive Storytelling:** Reading books becomes a communication adventure! Point to pictures, ask questions about the story, and encourage your child to participate by making sounds or using gestures to tell you what they think might happen next.

- **Augmentative and Alternative Communication (AAC):** Some children with Down syndrome might benefit from using AAC tools to supplement spoken communication. These can include picture boards, electronic devices with pre-recorded messages, or sign language. Talk to your speech therapist about exploring different AAC options.

Development

Every child develops at their own pace, and your child with Down syndrome is no exception. Here are some ways to support their development in a fun and nurturing way:

- **Early Intervention Programs:** Early intervention is key! These programs provide therapies like:

  - **Physical Therapy:** Helps develop gross motor skills like walking, running, and jumping, as well as fine motor skills like grasping objects and writing.

  - **Occupational Therapy:** Focuses on everyday skills like dressing, self-care, and participating in play activities.

  - **Speech Therapy:** Works on communication skills, including spoken language, understanding language, and using gestures and facial expressions effectively.

- **Sensory Integration:** Children with Down syndrome might have unique sensory preferences. A therapist can help you understand your child's sensory needs and create a calming or stimulating environment as needed.

- **The Magic of Routines:** Having a predictable routine provides comfort and security for your child. Establish routines for daily activities like mealtimes, playtime, and bedtime. This helps them anticipate what is coming next and feel more in control.

- **Learning Through Exploration:** Encourage your child to explore their environment safely. Provide them with a variety of toys and activities that promote motor skills, cognitive development, and problem-solving.

Self-Esteem

Self-esteem is the cornerstone of a happy and fulfilling life. Here are some ways to nurture your child's positive self-image:

- **Celebrating Strengths, Big and Small:** Make a point to celebrate your child's unique talents and abilities. This could be anything from memorizing their favorite song to mastering a new skill like building with Legos.

- **Positive Reinforcement:** When your child tries their best or accomplishes something new, shower them with praise and encouragement. Be specific about what they did well: "Wow, you worked so hard to build that tower! You are a great builder!"

- **The Power of "Yet":** When your child faces a challenge, use encouraging phrases like "You haven't figured it out yet, but I know you can do it with practice!" This instills a growth mindset and helps them persevere through difficulties.

- **Choice and Independence:** Whenever possible, offer your child choices. Even small choices, like picking out their clothes or choosing which toy to play with, empower them and build their confidence.

- **Modeling Positive Self-Talk:** Children learn by observing their parents. Be kind and patient with yourself, and celebrate your own accomplishments. Your positive self-talk will rub off on your child.

Remember, you are your child's biggest cheerleader. By focusing on communication, development, and self-esteem, you will be building a strong foundation that empowers your child to thrive. This chapter is just the beginning of your incredible journey together!

3. SUPPORTING YOUR FAMILY

Having a child with Down syndrome not only brings a whirlwind of emotions and excitement, but also concerns about how it might affect your other children and your family dynamic. This chapter is your guide to nurturing strong bonds between siblings and creating a supportive network that empowers your entire family to thrive.

Building Strong Sibling Bonds

Your children are embarking on a lifelong journey together – one filled with laughter, love, and unique challenges. Here are some ways to help them build a strong and lasting connection:

- **Involving Siblings Early On:** From the very beginning, include your other children in your child with Down syndrome's care routine in age-appropriate ways. Let them help with simple tasks like fetching toys or singing songs. This fosters a sense of responsibility, ownership, and strengthens the bond from a young age.

- **Celebrating Differences, Fostering Teamwork:** Help your children understand that everyone is unique, and Down syndrome is just one part of what makes their sibling special. Focus on their shared interests – maybe they both love building with blocks or reading stories. Encourage them to work together to build the biggest tower or act out their favorite characters.

- **Open Communication is Key:** Open and honest communication is essential. Talk openly with your children about Down syndrome, answer their questions honestly and age-appropriately, and create a safe space for them to express their feelings freely without judgment. You might answer your child's question about Down syndrome by saying, "Down syndrome means your sibling has an extra copy of a chromosome, which makes them special in their own way. They might learn things at a different pace, but that does not mean they can't learn amazing things!"

- **Creating Special Sibling Time:** Set aside dedicated time for your children to play together without distractions. It could be building forts in the living room, reading stories in a cozy nook, or playing a board game designed for all abilities. This dedicated time strengthens their bond, allows them to create happy memories, and teaches them valuable social skills like sharing and cooperation.

Creating a Support Network

Building a network of love and support will benefit your entire family. Connecting with others who understand your journey can offer guidance, encouragement, and a sense of belonging. Here are some ways to expand your support network:

- **Family and Friends:** Talk to your family and close friends about your child with Down syndrome. Share your hopes, concerns, and experiences. You might be surprised by the outpouring of love, understanding, and willingness to help. Consider inviting friends and family over for playdates or potlucks, allowing them to connect with your child with Down syndrome and build positive relationships.

- **Support Groups:** Connecting with other families who have children with Down syndrome is invaluable. These groups provide a safe space to share experiences, learn from each other, and build lasting friendships. You can find local support groups through hospitals, community centers, or online resources. Here, you can connect with families facing similar challenges, ask questions without judgment, and find emotional support.

- **Online Communities:** Online forums and social media groups can connect you with a wider network of families facing similar challenges. You can share tips, resources, and stories of inspiration. Online communities can be helpful for finding specific information, like strategies for managing challenging behaviors or recommendations for therapists and doctors.

Remember:

- **Sibling Rivalry is Normal:** Occasional sibling rivalry is a natural part of family life. Do not be discouraged if it arises. Talk to your children about sharing, patience, and the importance of being kind to one another. Equip them with tools for resolving conflicts peacefully, like using "I" statements and taking turns.

- **Self-Care is Essential:** Taking care of yourself is crucial. Schedule time for activities you enjoy, whether it is reading a book, taking a relaxing walk, or spending time with friends. A well-rested and happy parent is better equipped to manage the challenges of raising a child with Down syndrome and creates a more positive and stable environment for your entire family.

- **Celebrate Every Milestone:** Every achievement, big or small, is a reason to celebrate! Celebrate your children's successes, both individual and together, as a family. Celebrating strengthens family bonds, boosts self-esteem, and creates lasting positive memories.

This chapter is a roadmap to foster strong relationships within your family and build a supportive network outside it. Remember, you are not alone. With open communication, patience, and a whole lot of love, you can create a happy and fulfilling environment for your entire family.

4. NAVIGATING EDUCATION TOGETHER

The world of education is about to open its doors to your amazing child with Down syndrome! This chapter equips you with the knowledge and tools to navigate this exciting journey, ensuring inclusion and success in the classroom.

Understanding Your Options

Every child with Down syndrome learns differently. Here is a closer look at some common educational settings, each offering a unique approach to fostering your child's development:

- **General Education Classroom (with Support):** This option places your child in a regular classroom with typically developing peers. They will learn alongside their classmates, while receiving additional support from a special education teacher or instructional assistant. This support might involve:

  - **Differentiated Instruction:** Teachers may tailor lessons to meet your child's specific needs. This could include breaking down complex tasks into smaller steps, using visual aids, or providing one-on-one instruction during group activities.

- o **Assistive Technology:** Technology can be a powerful tool for learning. Your child might benefit from using devices like audiobooks, text-to-speech software, or specialized computer programs designed to support learning.

- **Resource Room:** This specialized setting provides small-group instruction for specific subjects or skills. Your child might attend the resource room for math, reading, or social skills development, while spending the remainder of the day in the general education classroom, interacting with their peers.

- **Self-Contained Classroom:** This structured environment offers intensive, individualized instruction delivered by a dedicated special education teacher. It is ideal for children who require significant support to access the curriculum and benefit from a highly structured learning environment.

The Power of Early Intervention

Starting early is crucial! Look for schools that offer Individualized Education Programs (IEPs).

- **IEPs:** These customized plans are like roadmaps for your child's education. They detail your child's unique strengths, needs, and goals. The IEP will outline:

  o **Present Levels of Performance (PLPs):** This section describes your child's current skills and abilities in different areas like reading, math, communication, and social interaction.

  o **Annual Goals:** These are specific, measurable objectives that your child will work towards throughout the school year.

  o **Special Education and Related Services:** This section outlines the support services your child will receive, such as speech therapy, occupational therapy, or physical therapy, to help them achieve their goals.

  o **Least Restrictive Environment (LRE):** This principle ensures your child is placed in the most inclusive setting possible, receiving support in the general education classroom whenever appropriate.

Collaborative Support for Your Child

Building a strong team around your child fosters a supportive and inclusive learning environment. Here are your key allies:

- **Special Education Teacher:** This dedicated educator collaborates with you and your child's general education teacher to develop and implement your child's IEP. They will provide specialized instruction, monitor your child's progress, and advocate for their needs within the school system.

- **General Education Teacher:** Your child's general education teacher plays a vital role in inclusion. Communicate openly with them about your child's needs and learning style. You can discuss strategies for modifying lessons, providing support in the classroom, and creating a welcoming environment for all students.

- **Therapists:** Speech therapists, occupational therapists, and physical therapists might provide additional support to address your child's specific needs. They will work with your child on improving communication skills, motor skills, and self-care abilities, all of which contribute to success in school.

Fostering Inclusion

Inclusion is about creating a welcoming and supportive environment where your child feels valued and can learn alongside their peers. Here are some ways to promote inclusion:

- **Self-Advocacy Skills:** As your child grows older, encourage them to become self-advocates. This means teaching them to communicate their needs and ask for help when they need it. Role-playing different scenarios can help your child practice self-advocacy skills in a safe and supportive environment.

- **Peer Support Programs:** These programs pair your child with typically developing peers who can offer friendship and support. This fosters social interaction, a sense of belonging, and a deeper understanding of one another.

- **Positive Classroom Environment:** A positive and accepting classroom environment is crucial. Talk to your child's teachers about strategies to create a welcoming space where diversity is celebrated. This might involve creating visuals that explain Down syndrome to classmates or incorporating activities that promote teamwork and understanding.

Remember

- **Be Your Child's Advocate:** You are your child's biggest champion! Do not hesitate to ask questions, advocate for your child's needs, and collaborate with their teachers to ensure they receive the best possible education. Familiarize yourself with the Individuals with Disabilities Education Act (IDEA), which guarantees your child's right to a free and appropriate public education (FAPE) in the least restrictive environment (LRE).

- **Celebrate Every Milestone:** Every accomplishment, big or small, deserves recognition! Celebrate your child's progress in school, no matter how big or small, to boost their confidence and motivation. Here are some specific examples you can celebrate: making a new friend, mastering a new skill like writing their name, or participating in a classroom activity.

- **Focus on Progress, Not Perfection:** Learning takes time and practice. Focus on your child's progress rather than achieving perfection. Every step forward is a victory! Maintain a positive attitude and celebrate your child's effort, even if they do not always get the answer right.

- **Communication is Key:** Open and honest communication between parents, teachers, and therapists is essential. Schedule regular meetings to discuss your child's progress, address any challenges, and celebrate their successes.

This chapter is just the beginning of your child's incredible educational journey. With a collaborative approach, an understanding of your options, and a focus on inclusion, you can help your child navigate the world of education with confidence and achieve their full potential. Remember, you are not alone on this journey. There are educators, therapists, and other families who can offer support and guidance along the way. Embrace the journey, celebrate the victories, and focus on the amazing things your child can accomplish!

5. HEALTHCARE & ADDRESSING SPECIFIC NEEDS

Your child with Down syndrome is a radiant bundle of joy, and keeping them healthy and happy is your top priority. This chapter dives into the world of healthcare for children with Down syndrome, focusing on building strong relationships with your child's medical team and addressing some common health concerns.

Building a Strong Doctor-Patient Relationship

Finding a healthcare provider you trust is the foundation for your child's well-being. Here are some ways to build a strong and collaborative relationship with your child's doctor:

- **Seek Recommendations:** Talk to other parents of children with Down syndrome or your child's pediatrician for recommendations. Look for doctors who are familiar with Down syndrome and have experience treating children with this condition. Consider factors like location, availability, and bedside manner when making your choice.

- **Open Communication is a Two-Way Street:** Be open and honest with your doctor about your child's health, from minor colds to developmental milestones. Do not be afraid to ask questions, no matter how small they may seem. The more information you share, the better your doctor can understand your child's unique needs.

- **Become a Partner in Care:** View your doctor as a partner, not just someone who tells you what to do. Come prepared to appointments with questions and concerns. Discuss treatment options together and make informed decisions about your child's healthcare journey.

Understanding Common Health Concerns

Children with Down syndrome might be more susceptible to certain health conditions. Here is a breakdown of some common concerns and how to address them proactively:

- **Hearing and Vision Problems:** Regular screenings for hearing and vision problems are crucial from a young age. Early detection and intervention are essential for optimal development. Schedule hearing tests with an audiologist and vision screenings with an ophthalmologist to identify any potential issues promptly.

- **Heart Conditions:** Congenital heart defects, meaning heart defects present at birth, are more common in children with Down syndrome.

Regular checkups with a cardiologist, a heart specialist, can help monitor any potential issues and ensure early intervention if needed.

- **Thyroid Issues:** The thyroid gland plays a vital role in metabolism and growth. Children with Down syndrome might be more prone to thyroid problems that can affect their development. Routine blood tests can help identify and manage any thyroid imbalances.

- **Sleep Apnea:** This condition can disrupt sleep patterns and lead to daytime fatigue. Symptoms include loud snoring and gasping for air during sleep. Talk to your doctor if you notice your child snoring heavily or having trouble sleeping through the night. A sleep study might be recommended to diagnose sleep apnea and determine appropriate treatment options.

- **Dental Concerns:** Regular dental checkups are important for maintaining good oral health. Children with Down syndrome might have smaller mouths and weaker jaw muscles, making them more prone to tooth decay and gum disease. Schedule regular appointments with a dentist familiar with caring for children with Down syndrome.

Remember

- **Early Intervention is Key:** The earlier any health concerns are detected and addressed, the better the outcome for your child. Do not hesitate to bring up any concerns you have with your doctor, no matter how small they may seem.

- **Regular Checkups:** Schedule regular checkups with your child's pediatrician and any specialists they might need to see. These checkups allow for early detection of any potential issues and ensure your child stays up-to-date on necessary vaccinations.

- **Healthy Habits:** Promote healthy habits like a balanced diet rich in fruits, vegetables, and whole grains, regular exercise appropriate for your child's age and abilities, and adequate sleep. These lifestyle choices contribute to a strong immune system and overall well-being.

Nurturing Emotional Wellbeing

Just like everyone else, children with Down syndrome experience a range of emotions. Here are some ways to support their emotional well-being:

- **Open Communication:** Create a safe space for your child to express their feelings, both positive and negative. Talk to them openly about their emotions and help them develop healthy coping mechanisms for dealing with frustration, anger, or sadness. This might involve using visuals like picture cards to represent emotions, role-playing scenarios, or teaching them simple relaxation techniques like deep breathing exercises.

- **Socialization is Key:** Encourage social interaction with other children. This can happen through playdates, joining a sports team, or participating in after-school activities. Socialization helps your child develop social skills, build friendships, and feel a sense of belonging.

- **Positive Reinforcement:** Celebrate your child's accomplishments, no matter how big or small. Focus on their strengths and encourage them to try new things. Positive reinforcement builds self-esteem and confidence, promoting emotional well-being.

Remember

- **Every Child is Unique:** While this chapter provides a general overview of common health concerns, it is important to remember that every child with Down syndrome is unique. The best approach is to work collaboratively with your child's doctor to develop a personalized healthcare plan that addresses their specific needs and preferences.

- **Advocacy is Empowering:** Do not be afraid to be your child's advocate. Learn as much as you can about Down syndrome and common health concerns. Ask questions, seek clarification, and participate actively in your child's healthcare decisions. There are many resources available online and through support groups to empower you as an advocate for your child.

- **The Importance of Support Systems:** Building a strong support system is crucial for your child's well-being and your own. Connect with other parents of children with Down syndrome, either online or through local support groups. Share experiences, offer encouragement to each other, and access valuable resources.

Looking Ahead

With proactive care, a strong support system, and a focus on healthy habits, you can empower your child to thrive and live a happy and healthy life! This chapter is just the beginning of your incredible journey together. Embrace the unique challenges and celebrate the remarkable milestones. Remember, your love, care, and unwavering support are the most powerful tools you have to help your child with Down syndrome blossom and reach their full potential.

6. DEVELOPING SOCIAL SKILLS

Your child with Down syndrome is a social butterfly, radiating warmth and eagerness to connect! This chapter equips you with strategies to nurture their social skills, cultivate confidence, and foster lasting friendships.

Understanding Social Development: A Spectrum of Strengths

Social development in children with Down syndrome can progress on a spectrum. Here is a breakdown of some key areas to focus on, keeping in mind your child's unique strengths and challenges:

- **Communication:** This encompasses both verbal and nonverbal communication. Encourage your child to express themselves using words, gestures, facial expressions, and even assistive technology like picture cards or communication apps. Play games that promote verbal skills like storytelling or charades. For nonverbal communication, help your child understand the importance of eye contact, facial expressions, and body language in conveying their message.

- **Turn-Taking and Sharing:** These are fundamental social skills for building friendships. Practice turn-taking with simple games like board games or taking turns pushing a swing. Use positive reinforcement, like praise or stickers, when your child successfully shares a toy or waits patiently for their turn.

- **Social Interaction:** Creating opportunities for your child to interact with other children is crucial. Consider enrolling them in age-appropriate activities like sports teams, after-school clubs, or drama classes. Organize playdates with children in their neighborhood or classmates.

Building Confidence

Confidence is the cornerstone of successful social interaction. Here are some ways to help your child blossom:

- **Positive Reinforcement:** Celebrate your child's efforts, big or small. This could be anything from trying a new food to mastering a new skill like putting on their shoes independently. Positive reinforcement builds self-esteem and motivates them to keep trying, even when faced with challenges.

- **Focus on Strengths:** Highlight your child's unique talents and abilities. This could be anything from their artistic abilities to their exceptional memory. Focusing on strengths builds confidence and allows them to shine in social settings.

- **Encourage Independence:** As your child grows, encourage them to do things for themselves whenever possible. This could be simple tasks like getting dressed, setting the table, or packing their backpack. Promoting independence builds confidence and a sense of accomplishment, which translates into a more positive social presence.

Fostering Friendships: Building Bridges of Connection

Friendships are essential for social development and emotional well-being. Here are some ways to help your child build lasting connections:

- **Playdates with Purpose:** Organize playdates with children of similar ages who share similar interests. This allows your child to practice social skills in a relaxed and supportive environment. Before the playdate, prepare your child by discussing potential activities and how to initiate play.

- **Social Skills Groups:** Consider enrolling your child in social skills groups specifically designed for children with Down syndrome. These groups provide a safe space to learn and practice social skills with peers facing similar challenges. Look for groups that incorporate activities tailored to your child's age and developmental level.

- **Positive Role Models:** Expose your child to positive role models with Down syndrome who are thriving in social settings. This can be through books, movies, or even meeting other children with Down syndrome involved in activities your child enjoys. Seeing positive examples can motivate your child and show them the possibilities for successful social interaction.

Remember

- **Patience is Key:** Developing social skills takes time and practice. Be patient with your child and celebrate their progress along the way. Focus on small victories, like initiating conversation with a peer or sharing a toy.

- **Embrace Differences:** Help your child understand that everyone is unique and has different strengths and weaknesses. Celebrate diversity and create opportunities for your child to interact with people from different backgrounds.

- **Open Communication:** Maintain open communication with your child about social interaction. Discuss challenges they might face, like difficulty understanding social cues or expressing themselves clearly. Role-play scenarios to help them develop strategies for overcoming these challenges.

Beyond the Chapter: A Journey of Connection and Growth

This chapter is a roadmap to fostering your child's social development and building lifelong friendships. Remember, every child is unique, and social development happens at their own pace. With encouragement, patience, and a focus on building confidence, you can help your child blossom into a socially adept and well-adjusted individual. Embrace the journey, celebrate the victories, and watch your child build meaningful connections that enrich their lives!

7. LEISURE & INDEPENDENCE

Your child with Down syndrome is a ball of sunshine, brimming with energy and a zest for life! This chapter explores two vital aspects of their journey: nurturing their passions through engaging leisure activities and planning for a future filled with independence.

Exploring Passions

Leisure activities are not just fun and games; they play a crucial role in a child's development. Here are some ways to help your child discover and explore their passions:

- **Expose Them to a Kaleidoscope of Activities:** Provide opportunities to try a variety of activities, venturing beyond the typical. This could include team sports like soccer or basketball, individual activities like swimming or gymnastics, or creative pursuits like music lessons, art classes, or cooking workshops. Consider options like drama clubs, robotics teams, or even volunteering at an animal shelter. The wider the range of experiences, the more likely your child is to discover something that truly sparks their joy.

- **Focus on Strengths and Spark New Interests:** Build upon your child's existing strengths and natural inclinations. If they have a rhythmic soul, enroll them in a drumming class. If they possess a keen eye for detail, introduce them to model building or photography. Do not be afraid to introduce new activities that might pique their curiosity. You might discover a hidden talent for playing the guitar or a newfound passion for coding!

- **The Magic of Play: Learning Through Laughter:** Play is a natural language for children, a way for them to learn and explore the world around them. Engage in playful activities together – build elaborate castles with blocks, put on a puppet show fueled by imagination, or have a dance party in the living room. This fosters a love for learning and exploration, all while strengthening the bond between you and your child.

Developing Independence

As your child matures, fostering independence empowers them to confidently navigate their world. Here are some ways to help them develop essential life skills:

- **Start Early, Start Simple:** Begin with age-appropriate tasks like setting the table for dinner, sorting laundry by color, or making their bed.

Break down complex tasks into smaller, manageable steps and provide support as needed. As your child masters these tasks, gradually increase the complexity, introducing new responsibilities like packing a lunchbox or helping with simple household chores.

- **Practice Makes Perfect: Cultivating Confidence Through Repetition** The more your child practices a skill, the more confident they become. Encourage them to do things for themselves, even if it takes longer or requires some initial assistance. Celebrate their efforts and acknowledge their progress, no matter how small. Positive reinforcement builds confidence and motivates them to keep trying.

- **Communication is Key: A Roadmap to Success** Open communication is crucial. Talk to your child about their goals for independence and work together to create a plan. Listen to their concerns and address any challenges they might face. Role-playing scenarios can be a helpful tool, allowing your child to practice real-life situations in a safe and supportive environment.

Planning for the Future

Thinking about the future can feel daunting, but

proactive planning sets your child up for success. Here are some key areas to consider:

- **Education: Unveiling Paths to Lifelong Learning** Discuss options for post-secondary education or vocational training programs that align with your child's interests and skills. Explore possibilities like community colleges offering certificate programs in specific trades, or specialized programs designed for individuals with Down syndrome that focus on independent living skills and career development.

- **Independent Living: Building a Nest for a Thriving Adult** Research options for supported living arrangements or independent living skills programs. These programs can empower your child to live a fulfilling and independent life as an adult, providing them with the necessary support and resources to thrive.

- **Financial Security: Investing in a Secure Future** Start planning for your child's financial future early on. Explore options like trusts or supported employment programs that can help them achieve financial independence. Talk to a financial advisor to create a personalized plan that meets your child's specific needs and goals.

Remember

- **Individualized Approach: Tailoring the Journey to Your Child's Needs** Every child develops at their own pace and has unique strengths and interests. Tailor your approach to fostering leisure and independence to your child's individual needs and strengths. There is no one-size-fits-all approach!

- **Celebrate Milestones, Big and Small: Acknowledgement Fuels Growth** No matter how big or small, celebrate your child's achievements. This could be anything from mastering a new recipe to participating in a new activity for the first time. Recognition and positive reinforcement fuel their motivation and confidence.

- **The Power of Support: Building a Network for Success** Building a network of support is crucial for both you and your child. Connect with other parents of children with Down syndrome, either online or through local support groups. Share experiences, offer encouragement to each other, and access valuable resources. Consider collaborating with educators, therapists, and social workers to create a comprehensive plan that supports your child's development and future goals.

Beyond the Chapter: A Journey of Exploration and Empowerment

This chapter is just the beginning of your child's incredible journey towards discovering their passions and achieving independence. Embrace the process, celebrate the victories, and watch your child blossom into a confident and capable individual, ready to embrace the world with all its possibilities! Remember, your unwavering love, support, and guidance are the most powerful tools you have to empower your child to reach their full potential and live a happy, fulfilling life.

8. THE JOYS AND CHALLENGES

The arrival of your child with Down syndrome marks a momentous occasion, a whirlwind of emotions filled with both joy and wonder. This chapter explores the beautiful spectrum of feelings that come with raising a child with Down syndrome, equipping you to navigate challenges with grace and celebrate victories with immense pride.

A Kaleidoscope of Emotions

The emotions you experience as a parent of a child with Down syndrome are vast and varied, like a kaleidoscope reflecting a multitude of colors. Here is a breakdown of some common feelings:

- **Overwhelming Joy:** Witnessing your child's milestones, their contagious laughter, and their pure, unadulterated love can fill your heart with a joy that overflows. Celebrate these moments, big and small, from the first gummy grin to the first wobbly steps. They are precious treasures to be cherished and woven into the fabric of your family's story.

- **Fear and Uncertainty:** The unknown can be a daunting landscape. You might worry about your child's future, their health, or their ability to navigate the world independently. These anxieties are perfectly normal. Remember, you are not alone. There are resources and support systems available to help you navigate these uncertainties. Talk to your pediatrician, connect with other parents, and do not hesitate to seek professional guidance if needed.

- **Frustration and Impatience:** There will be times when progress feels slow, or challenges arise that test your patience. Perhaps your child struggles with learning a new skill, or communication feels like a frustrating puzzle. It is okay to feel frustrated or impatient. Take a deep breath, seek support from your network, and remember that every child develops at their own pace. Celebrate the small victories, like mastering a new step in a self-care routine or finally grasping a new concept.

- **Pride and Accomplishment:** Witnessing your child overcome challenges, learn new skills, and blossom into their unique personality will fill you with immense pride. It might be the first time they successfully tie their shoes, the day they deliver a clear and concise sentence, or the moment they confidently participate in a group activity. Celebrate their accomplishments, no matter how small, and acknowledge the effort they put in. Your encouragement will fuel their motivation and sense of self-worth.

Transforming Obstacles into Opportunities

While there might be challenges, they can also be opportunities for growth and learning. Here are some ways to approach them:

- **Early Intervention is Key:** Early intervention programs can significantly improve your child's development and quality of life. These programs often involve a team of specialists, like speech therapists, occupational therapists, and physical therapists, working together to address your child's specific needs. Talk to your pediatrician about available options and access to specialists.

- **Building a Support System:** Connect with other parents of children with Down syndrome, either online or through local support groups. Share experiences, offer encouragement to each other, and access valuable resources. Support groups can be a lifeline, providing a sense of community and understanding. You can learn from each other's successes and challenges, and forge lasting friendships built on shared experiences.

- **Advocacy is Empowering:** Become your child's champion. Learn as much as you can about Down syndrome, common health concerns, and available resources. Be your child's advocate, speaking up for their needs and ensuring they receive the best possible care and education. Do not be afraid to ask questions, seek clarification, and participate actively in your child's healthcare decisions.

Celebrating the Joys

The journey of raising a child with Down syndrome is filled with countless joys, a symphony of love and laughter. Here are some ways to embrace them:

- **Focus on Strengths:** Every child has unique strengths and talents. Perhaps your child has a natural artistic ability, a knack for music, or an infectious enthusiasm for sports. Celebrate your child's individuality and encourage them to pursue their passions. Whether it is painting vibrant landscapes, mastering a new musical instrument, or participating in an adaptive sports league, nurture their talents and watch them shine.

- **The Power of Play:** Play is essential for all children, but especially for children with Down syndrome. Engage in playful activities together, fostering a bond and creating lasting memories.

From building elaborate block towers to playing board games designed for social interaction, let your imaginations run wild. Laughter is a universal language, and playful moments create a foundation for connection and joy.

1. **Living in the Moment:** Savor the present moments. Witnessing your child's infectious laughter, their unconditional love, and their pure joy for life is a gift to be cherished. Put away distractions, be present in the moment, and create lasting memories together. Whether it is baking cookies in the kitchen, having a picnic in the park, or snuggling up for a bedtime story, cherish these everyday moments of connection and love.

Remember

- **Love is the Foundation:** Above all else, unconditional love is the foundation for your child's emotional well-being and development. Shower them with love, celebrate their individuality, and be their biggest cheerleader. Your unwavering love will create a safe and secure environment where they can thrive and reach their full potential.

- **Embrace the Journey:** The journey of raising a child with Down syndrome is unique and beautiful, child with Down syndrome is unique and beautiful, filled with twists and turns, laughter and tears. Embrace the challenges and celebrate the victories, one step at a time. There will be moments of frustration, but the unconditional love you share will create an unbreakable bond.

- **You Are Not Alone:** A strong support system is crucial. Connect with other parents, educators, and professionals who can offer guidance and understanding. There are many resources available online and through local organizations. Remember, you are not alone on this incredible journey. Together, you can create a world of love, acceptance, and opportunity for your child.

Beyond the Chapter: A Tapestry Woven with Love and Acceptance

This chapter is a mere glimpse into the beautiful and complex world of raising a child with Down syndrome. With love, acceptance, and a supportive network, you can navigate the challenges, celebrate the victories, and watch your child blossom into a happy, confident, and fulfilled individual. Embrace the full spectrum of emotions, for they all contribute to the incredible tapestry of your family's story. As your child grows, so will your love, your understanding, and your pride. The journey ahead is filled with possibilities, and together, you can create a future brimming with love, laughter, and endless possibilities.

9. BUILDING SUPPORTIVE NETWORKS AND SHARING EXPERIENCES

The arrival of your precious child with Down syndrome brings immense joy, but you might also wonder where to begin? This chapter dives into the importance of building a supportive community, a network of individuals who can become your guiding stars, offering encouragement, practical advice, and a profound sense of belonging.

The Power of Connection

As you embark on this incredible adventure of raising a child with Down syndrome, remember that you are not alone. There is a vast and vibrant world of support waiting to be discovered. Building a strong community offers a multitude of benefits:

- **Shared Experiences: A Balm for the Soul** Connecting with other parents who understand the unique joys and challenges of raising a child with Down syndrome can be incredibly validating. You can share stories, ask questions without judgment, and offer encouragement to each other. Hearing success stories from other families can be a powerful motivator during difficult times.

- **A Wealth of Knowledge: Tapping into a Reservoir of Expertise** Seasoned parents and professionals within the Down syndrome community are a treasure trove of knowledge. They can share valuable resources on topics like navigating therapies, exploring educational options, or tackling common behavioral challenges. Their insights, gleaned from personal experience, can provide a roadmap for your own journey.

- **Emotional Support: A Safe Space to Share Your Heart** There will be times when you face hurdles or simply need a listening ear. A supportive community provides a safe haven to express your emotions, vent frustrations without judgment, and celebrate victories, big or small. Knowing you have a network of understanding individuals to lean on can significantly reduce stress and bolster your emotional well-being.

Where to Find Support

There are many avenues to explore as you connect with others in the Down syndrome community. Here are some starting points:

- **Online Support Groups: A Global Network at Your Fingertips** Join online forums or social media groups specifically dedicated to Down syndrome. These platforms allow you to connect with parents from all over the world, fostering a sense of global community. You can share experiences, offer support, and gain valuable insights from the comfort of your home.

- **Local Organizations: Building Connections in Your Backyard** Many cities and towns have local Down syndrome organizations that offer a variety of resources, including support groups, workshops, and even family events. Connecting with these organizations allows you to build a local support network and forge meaningful relationships with families in your area facing similar experiences.

- **Therapists and Educators: Partners on Your Child's Journey** Your child's therapists and educators can be valuable resources for building your support network. They might be aware of local support groups or programs specifically designed for families raising children with Down syndrome. Do not hesitate to ask them for recommendations or guidance in connecting with the broader community.

Building Meaningful Connections

Here are some practical tips to help you build strong and meaningful connections within your community:

- **Be Open and Approachable: Letting Your Light Shine** Let others know you are interested in connecting. Strike up conversations with other parents at therapy appointments, or participate actively in online forums. Do not be afraid to initiate conversations and share your story.

- **Be an Active Listener: The Power of Empathy** Show genuine interest in others' experiences and challenges. Listen attentively, offer words of encouragement, and ask thoughtful questions to demonstrate your understanding.

- **Respect Differences: Celebrating Diversity Within the Community** Remember, every child with Down syndrome develops at their own pace and has unique strengths and needs. Be respectful of these differences and celebrate the diversity within the community. Embrace the fact that each family's journey is unique.

- **Give Back and Share Your Experiences: The Ripple Effect of Support** As you gain knowledge and experience, consider offering support to others who are new to the journey. Share your experiences, offer advice, and be a source of encouragement for others. By giving back, you strengthen the entire community and create a ripple effect of support.

Remember

- **Building a community takes time.** Do not get discouraged if it takes time to find your perfect circle of support. Be patient and persistent in your efforts, and eventually, you will find your tribe.

- **The right connections make a difference.** The people you surround yourself with can significantly impact your journey. Seek out positive, supportive, and inspiring individuals who uplift you and celebrate your victories.

- **You are part of something bigger.** By building a community, you are not just creating a support network for yourself, but also for others. Together, you can create a more inclusive and supportive world for children with Down syndrome, fostering acceptance and understanding.

Beyond the Chapter: A Journey of Shared Strength and Unwavering Support

This chapter is just the beginning of your journey towards building a strong and supportive community. Remember, the connections you forge can be a source of immense strength and encouragement. With a supportive network by your side, you can face challenges with confidence, celebrate victories with joy, and create a fulfilling and enriching life for your child. So, embrace the power of connection, reach out, and build a community that will empower you on this incredible journey.

Building Bridges with Professionals

Your support network should extend beyond fellow parents. Here are some key professionals to connect with:

- **Doctors and Specialists:** Pediatricians, developmental pediatricians, geneticists, and other specialists can provide vital medical care and guidance specific to your child's needs. Building a strong relationship with these professionals allows them to provide comprehensive care and address any health concerns that might arise.

- **Therapists:** Speech therapists, occupational therapists, physical therapists, and behavioral therapists can play a crucial role in your child's development. These professionals can work with your child to improve their communication skills, motor skills, and overall well-being.

- **Educators:** Teachers, special education specialists, and inclusion specialists can help ensure your child receives a quality education tailored to their individual needs. Collaborating with educators and advocating for your child's rights within the school system is essential for their academic success and social integration.

Fostering Inclusive Relationships

As you navigate the world with your child, you might encounter individuals who lack understanding of Down syndrome. Here are some ways to promote inclusivity:

- **Embrace Opportunities to Educate:** If someone expresses curiosity or asks questions about Down syndrome, take it as an opportunity to educate them. Briefly explain the condition, highlight your child's strengths, and advocate for acceptance.

- **Challenge Stereotypes:** Gently correct any misconceptions or stereotypes you encounter. Promote a positive image of Down syndrome and focus on your child's unique personality and abilities.

- **Celebrate Differences:** Embrace the fact that everyone is unique, and differences should be celebrated. Create opportunities for your child to interact with typically developing children, fostering friendships and understanding.

Remember

- **You Are Your Child's Advocate:** Be your child's voice and champion. Speak up for their needs, ensure they receive appropriate support, and advocate for a world that embraces inclusivity and celebrates diversity.

- **The Journey is a Marathon, Not a Sprint:** Building a strong community takes time and effort. Be patient, persistent, and celebrate the connections you forge along the way.

- **Together We Are Stronger:** By sharing experiences, offering support, and working together, the Down syndrome community can create a more inclusive and supportive world for all.

Beyond the Chapter: A Tapestry Woven with Love and Support

This chapter has explored the importance of building a supportive community. Remember, the connections you build can become the threads that weave a beautiful tapestry of love, support, and shared experiences. With a strong community by your side, you can face any challenge, celebrate every victory, and create a fulfilling and enriching life for your child. So, embrace the power of connection, reach out, and build a community that will empower you and your child on this incredible journey.

10. UNDERSTANDING SENSORY PROCESSING

Imagine your child's world as a vibrant symphony of sights, sounds, smells, tastes, and textures. This chapter explores the concept of sensory processing, how it can differ in children with Down syndrome, and ways to support your child with love and understanding.

The Wonderful World of Senses

Our senses are like doorways to the world around us. They allow us to experience sight, sound, smell, taste, touch, movement (vestibular system), body awareness (proprioception), and internal sensations (interoception). Our brains process this sensory information and help us understand our environment.

Sensory Processing: When the Symphony Gets Out of Tune

Sometimes, the brain has difficulty processing sensory information. This is called sensory processing disorder (SPD). Children with Down syndrome may experience SPD, which can affect how they interact with their environment.

Here are some ways SPD might manifest:

- **Oversensitivity:** Certain sights, sounds, smells, or textures might feel overwhelming or unpleasant. For example, loud noises might be painful, or bright lights might cause discomfort.

- **Under-sensitivity:** Your child might not seem to register certain sensations. For instance, they might not feel pain as readily, or they might crave strong sensory input like loud noises or rough textures.

- **Sensory Seeking:** Your child might actively seek out specific sensory experiences. They might crave movement, jump on furniture, or spin in circles.

Understanding Your Child's Sensory Needs

Every child experiences the world differently. Here is how to understand your child's unique sensory needs:

- **Observe and Respond:** Pay attention to your child's reactions to different sensory stimuli. Notice what seems to calm or upset them.

- **Open Communication:** As your child grows, talk to them about how they experience sensations. Encourage them to express their preferences and any discomfort they might feel.

- **Seek Professional Guidance:** If you suspect your child has SPD, consult a therapist or occupational therapist who specializes in sensory processing. They can provide a professional evaluation and recommend strategies to support your child.

Supporting Your Child with Love

There are many ways to create a loving and supportive environment that addresses your child's sensory needs:

- **Sensory Modifications:** Make adjustments in your daily routine to minimize overwhelming sensory input. Dim lights in certain areas, use noise-canceling headphones, or offer calming textures like soft blankets.

- **Sensory Activities:** Provide opportunities for your child to explore sensations in a safe and controlled way. Offer activities with different textures, play calming music, or create a sensory bin filled with interesting objects.

- **Positive Reinforcement:** Focus on praising your child's efforts to manage sensory input. Celebrate their progress and successes, no matter how small.

Remember

- **Every Child is Unique:** There is no one-size-fits-all approach to sensory processing. What works for one child might not work for another. Be patient and find what works best for your child.

- **Focus on Communication:** Open communication is key. The better you understand your child's sensory needs, the better you can support them.

- **Celebrate Differences:** Sensory processing differences are not something to be ashamed of. Embrace your child's unique way of experiencing the world.

Beyond the Chapter: A Journey of Understanding and Love

This chapter has explored the concept of sensory processing and how it might affect your child with Down syndrome. Remember, supporting your child's sensory needs is a journey of love and understanding. By creating a supportive environment, celebrating their individuality, and seeking professional guidance when needed, you can help your child navigate their sensory world with confidence. Together, you can create a beautiful symphony of love and acceptance.

11. PROMOTING HEALTHY HABITS

Imagine your child as a budding tree – healthy habits are like sunshine and water, nourishing them to grow strong and healthy. This chapter explores the importance of good nutrition, regular exercise, and quality sleep for children with Down syndrome. By providing a foundation of healthy habits, you will be nurturing your child's overall well-being for a lifetime.

Nutrition

Just like any plant needs the right nutrients to grow, our bodies need healthy foods to function properly. Here is why good nutrition is important for children with Down syndrome:

- **Energy Levels:** Eating a balanced diet provides your child with the energy they need to play, learn, and explore the world.

- **Physical Development:** Nutritious foods support healthy growth and development of muscles and bones.

- **Overall Health:** Good nutrition helps maintain a strong immune system, which fights off illnesses.

Building a Balanced Plate

Here are some tips for creating a balanced and healthy diet for your child:

- **Variety is Key:** Offer a rainbow of fruits and vegetables with different colors and textures. This ensures your child gets different vitamins and minerals.

- **Focus on Whole Foods:** Whole grains, lean protein sources like fish and chicken, and healthy fats like those found in avocados and nuts are essential for a balanced diet.

- **Limit Processed Foods:** Sugary drinks, processed snacks, and fast food are high in calories and low in nutrients. Limit these in your child's diet.

- **Fun and Engaging Meals:** Make mealtimes fun and engaging! Let your child help with age-appropriate tasks like setting the table or choosing a healthy snack.

Exercise

Just like sunshine helps a plant grow strong, regular exercise keeps our bodies healthy. Here is why exercise is important for children with Down syndrome:

- **Strength and Coordination:** Exercise builds muscle strength and improves motor skills like coordination and balance.

- **Weight Management:** Regular physical activity helps maintain a healthy weight, which is beneficial for overall health.

- **Feeling Good:** Exercise releases endorphins, which have mood-boosting effects and promote feelings of well-being.

Finding Fun Activities

There are many ways to incorporate exercise into your child's routine:

- **Family Activities:** Make physical activity a family affair! Go for walks, bike rides, or play tag in the park together.

- **Sports and Activities:** Encourage your child to participate in sports teams or activities they enjoy, like swimming, dance classes, or gymnastics.

- **Active Play at Home:** Even simple activities like playing active video games or dancing to music can get your child moving.

Sleep

Just like a plant needs darkness to rest and grow, a good night's sleep is crucial for our bodies to recharge. Here is why sleep is important for children with Down syndrome:

- **Brain Development:** Sleep allows the brain to consolidate learning and memories from the day.

- **Physical Growth:** During sleep, the body repairs itself and releases hormones essential for growth.

- **Emotional Well-Being:** A good night's sleep helps regulate emotions and promotes a positive mood.

Creating a Sleep Routine

Here are some tips for creating a relaxing bedtime routine:

- **Establish a Consistent Schedule:** Go to bed and wake up at similar times each day, even on weekends.

- **Calming Activities:** Wind down for bedtime with calming activities like reading a book, taking a warm bath, or listening to soothing music.

- **Create a Relaxing Environment:** Make sure your child's bedroom is dark, quiet, and cool for optimal sleep.

Remember

- **Start Early:** Developing healthy habits is easier when you start early on. Introduce healthy food choices, regular exercise, and a good sleep routine as soon as possible.

- **Be Patient and Consistent:** Building healthy habits takes time and patience. Be consistent with your approach and celebrate your child's progress along the way.

- **Make it a Family Affair:** Encourage healthy habits for the whole family. This sets a positive example for your child and creates a supportive environment.

Beyond the Chapter: A Journey of Growth and Well-Being

This chapter has explored the importance of promoting healthy habits for your child with Down syndrome. Remember, fostering healthy habits is a lifelong journey. By providing a foundation of good nutrition, regular exercise, and quality sleep, you will be nurturing the essential elements needed for your child to flourish and experience a lifetime of wellbeing. Just like a strong tree weathers storms and thrives through sunshine, your child will develop the resilience and well-being needed to navigate life's challenges and embrace all the possibilities that lie ahead.

12. POSITIVE BEHAVIOR MANAGEMENT

Imagine your child as a beautiful garden – flourishing with potential, yet sometimes requiring gentle guidance. This chapter explores positive behavior management strategies, helping you cultivate a loving and supportive environment where your child with Down syndrome can thrive.

Understanding Behavior

Before diving into strategies, it is crucial to understand why children with Down syndrome might exhibit challenging behaviors. Here are some common reasons:

- **Communication Difficulties:** Sometimes, frustration with limited communication skills can lead to outbursts or tantrums. Your child might be struggling to express their needs or wants.

- **Sensory Processing Issues:** As explored in a previous chapter, sensory processing differences can be overwhelming for your child. They might act out as a way to cope with these sensory challenges.

- **Seeking Attention:** Sometimes, challenging behavior might be a way for your child to get your attention, even if it is negative attention.

Building on Positive Reinforcement

Traditional punishment-based approaches might not be as effective with children with Down syndrome. Here is why positive behavior management is key:

- **Focus on the Positive:** Positive reinforcement focuses on rewarding desired behaviors, encouraging your child to repeat them. This fosters a more positive and productive learning environment.

- **Building Strong Bonds:** Positive interactions create strong bonds of trust and love between you and your child. This foundation makes it easier to work together on behavior management.

- **Understanding the Cause:** By addressing the underlying cause of the behavior, you can help your child learn positive alternatives for expression.

Effective Strategies to Nurture Your Child's Growth

Here are some positive behavior management strategies you can use:

- **Visual Aids:** Pictures, charts, and schedules can help your child understand expectations and routines. Visual cues can be especially helpful for children who learn best visually.

- **Positive Reinforcement:** When your child exhibits desired behavior, praise them! Offer verbal praise, hugs, high fives, or a small reward system to encourage positive choices.

- **Providing Choices:** Whenever possible, offer your child choices. This empowers them and reduces frustration. For example, "Do you want to wear the blue shirt or the green shirt?"

- **Redirection:** If your child is engaging in an unwanted behavior, gently redirect them to a more appropriate activity. Offer alternatives or suggest a calming activity.

- **Stay Calm and Consistent:** When faced with challenging behavior, stay calm and patient. Remain consistent with your expectations and responses.

Building Strong Foundation for Positive Behavior

Positive behavior management goes beyond just the strategies. Here is how to build a strong foundation for success:

- **Open Communication:** Create a safe space for open communication. Encourage your child to express their feelings and needs.

- **Quality Time:** Spend quality time with your child every day. Engage in activities they enjoy, fostering a loving and supportive connection.

- **Celebrate Milestones:** Celebrate even small victories in your child's behavior management journey. Acknowledge their progress and keep them motivated.

Remember

- **Every Child is Unique:** The best strategies will vary depending on your child's individual needs and personality. Be patient and experiment to find what works best for your family.

- **Seek Professional Guidance:** Do not hesitate to seek professional guidance from a therapist or behavior specialist if you are struggling with challenging behaviors.

- **Love is the Key:** Always remember, love and understanding are the cornerstones of positive behavior management. By nurturing a loving bond with your child, you will create a foundation for them to learn, grow, and thrive.

Beyond the Chapter: A Journey of Growth and Love

This chapter has equipped you with tools and strategies for positive behavior management. Remember, fostering positive behavior is a journey, not a destination. By building strong bonds, focusing on positive reinforcement, and seeking help when needed, you can cultivate a loving and supportive environment where your child with Down syndrome can flourish and reach their full potential.

13. TRANSITION PLANNING

Imagine your child as a hot air balloon, ready to soar to new heights. This chapter explores transition planning, the process of preparing your child with Down syndrome for different stages of life, equipping them with the tools they need to reach their full potential. By planning with love and foresight, you can help them navigate future transitions smoothly and confidently.

Transition Planning for Success

Transition planning might seem far off, but it is never too early to start. Here is why it is important:

- **Preparing for Independence:** As your child grows, they will naturally yearn for more independence. Transition planning helps them develop the skills needed to live, work, and navigate life as independently as possible.

- **Empowerment and Confidence:** Being prepared for future transitions fosters a sense of empowerment and confidence in your child.

- **A Smooth Journey:** Transitioning from school to work, living at home to living independently –

these can be life-altering events. Planning helps ensure a smooth and positive experience.

Stages of Transition

Here are some key stages where transition planning plays a crucial role:

- **From Early Intervention to School:** As your child transitions from early intervention programs to school, planning ensures a smooth entry and helps them adapt to the new environment.

- **School to Adulthood:** The transition from high school to adult life is a significant one. Planning helps your child explore vocational options, develop independent living skills, and prepare for potential further education.

- **Throughout Life:** Transition planning is not a one-time event. As your child navigates life, there will be ongoing transitions like moving jobs or living arrangements. Having a plan and support system in place eases these adjustments.

Planning with Love: A Journey Together

Here are some steps to take on your transition planning

journey:

- **Start Early:** Begin planning conversations early on, even if your child is young. As they mature, involve them in the planning process as much as possible.

- **Identify Goals:** Work with your child, teachers, therapists, and other professionals to identify goals for each stage of transition.

- **Develop a Plan:** Create a plan outlining the skills your child needs to develop, the resources available, and the steps you will take to support them.

- **Seek Professional Guidance:** Do not hesitate to seek help from transition specialists, social workers, or career counselors. They can provide valuable guidance and support.

Remember:

- **Focus on Strengths:** Build on your child's strengths and interests when planning for their future. Help them discover their passions and explore careers or living arrangements that align with them.

- **Celebrate Milestones:** As your child reaches milestones in their transition journey, celebrate their successes! This positive reinforcement keeps them motivated.

- **Flexibility is Key:** Life can be unpredictable. Be flexible and adaptable in your planning. Review and adjust your strategies as needed.

Beyond the Chapter: A Journey of Love and Support

This chapter has opened the door to transition planning. Remember, preparing your child for the future is a journey of love and support. By starting early, working together, and seeking help when needed, you can launch your child with Down syndrome into a bright future filled with possibilities. You will be their anchor, guiding them with love as they take flight and navigate life's exciting journey.

14. FINANCIAL CONSIDERATIONS

Imagine your child as a precious treasure you want to protect and nurture for life. This chapter explores the financial considerations for families caring for a loved one with Down syndrome. By planning with love and foresight, you can ensure your child's financial security and well-being throughout their journey.

Understanding the Unique Needs and Potential Challenges

Children with Down syndrome may have unique needs that impact your finances. Here is why financial planning is crucial:

- **Potential for Increased Medical Expenses:** People with Down syndrome might require ongoing medical care or therapy, leading to higher healthcare costs.

- **Long-Term Care Considerations:** As your child ages, they might require long-term care services, which can be expensive.

- **Government Benefits and Resources:** Several government benefits and resources are available to support individuals with disabilities.

Understanding these programs is vital for financial planning.

Planning for the Future: Building a Secure Foundation

Here are some key steps to take on your financial planning journey:

- **Early Planning is Key:** The sooner you start planning, the more time your money has to grow. This allows you to build a stronger financial foundation for your child's future.

- **Explore Government Benefits:** Research and apply for government benefits like Supplemental Security Income (SSI) or Medicaid, which can help offset medical and living expenses.

- **Consider Special Needs Trusts:** A special needs trust can hold assets for your child without jeopardizing their eligibility for government benefits. Talk to a financial advisor about setting up a trust.

- **Life Insurance:** Life insurance can provide financial security for your child in case you are no longer there. Explore different life insurance options and choose one that fits your needs.

- **Budgeting and Saving:** Develop a realistic budget and prioritize saving for your child's future. Even small amounts saved regularly can grow significantly over time.

Additional Resources: Seeking Guidance and Support

There are resources available to help you navigate financial planning for your child with Down syndrome:

- **Financial Advisors:** A financial advisor specializing in special needs can provide personalized guidance and recommend investment strategies.

- **Social Workers:** Social workers can connect you with government programs and resources that can benefit your child.

- **Support Groups:** Connecting with other families caring for loved ones with Down syndrome can provide valuable emotional and informational support.

Remember:

- **Knowledge is Power:** Educate yourself about financial resources and government benefits available to individuals with disabilities.

- **Open Communication:** Talk openly with your child about finances as they grow older. Empower them to understand and manage their finances as much as possible.

- **Peace of Mind:** By planning and preparing financially, you can gain peace of mind knowing you've taken steps to secure your child's future.

Beyond the Chapter: A Journey of Love and Security

This chapter has equipped you with knowledge and tools for financial planning. Remember, safeguarding your child's financial well-being is a journey of love and security. By starting early, seeking guidance, and making informed decisions, you can build a strong financial foundation, allowing your child to focus on living a fulfilling and secure life. You will be their guiding light, illuminating the path towards a brighter financial future.

15. LEGAL ISSUES AND FUTURE CONSIDERATIONS

Imagine your child as a beautiful garden, flourishing with potential, yet needing careful tending to ensure its long-term health. This chapter explores legal issues faced by families caring for a loved one with Down syndrome. By planning with love and foresight, you can create a legal framework that protects and nurtures your child's future well-being.

Understanding Legal Considerations

Life can be unpredictable. Legal planning helps ensure your child is cared for and their wishes are respected, even if you are no longer there. Here is why it is important:

- **Guardianship:** A guardian makes decisions about your child's care and finances if they are unable to do so themselves. Planning guardianship ensures someone you trust will make these important decisions.

- **Estate Planning:** Estate planning involves creating a plan for managing your assets after you pass away. This can include a will and trusts, which can benefit your child.

- **Future Considerations:** As your child grows older, legal documents like healthcare directives may be needed to outline their wishes for medical care.

Guardianship

A guardian is a trusted individual who makes legal and financial decisions for your child if they are unable to do so themselves. Here is what to consider when choosing a guardian:

- **Someone You Trust:** Choose someone who loves your child, understands their needs, and will act in their best interests.

- **Considering Age and Ability:** Select someone young enough and healthy enough to fulfill their role for the foreseeable future.

- **Discussing Your Wishes:** Talk openly with your chosen guardian about your expectations and your child's needs.

Estate Planning

Estate planning ensures your assets are distributed according to your wishes after you pass away. Here is how it can benefit your child:

- **Wills:** A will outlines who inherits your assets after you die. You can include specific bequests for your child.

- **Special Needs Trusts:** A special needs trust can hold assets for your child without jeopardizing their eligibility for government benefits. This can provide for their future needs without impacting their current support system.

Future Considerations: Empowering Your Child's Voice

As your child grows older, consider these additional legal steps:

- **Healthcare Directives:** A healthcare directive allows your child to specify their wishes for medical care in case they are unable to communicate them.

- **Power of Attorney:** A power of attorney allows your child to designate someone they trust to make financial decisions on their behalf if needed.

Remember

- **Start Early:** Do not wait until later in life to address legal issues. Starting early allows for thoughtful planning and avoids potential complications.

- **Seek Professional Guidance:** Consult with an attorney specializing in estate planning and special needs to create a legal plan that meets your child's specific needs.

- **Open Communication:** Talk openly with your child about your plans as they mature. This fosters trust and empowers them to understand their future options.

Beyond the Chapter: A Journey of Love and Protection

This chapter has equipped you with knowledge about legal considerations. Remember, protecting your child's future through legal planning is a journey of love and foresight. By taking proactive steps and seeking professional guidance, you can create a legal framework that safeguards your child's well-being and empowers them to navigate life's journey with confidence. You will be their nurturing gardener, ensuring their garden continues to flourish for years to come.

16. FOSTERING CREATIVITY

Imagine your child as a vibrant paintbrush, brimming with potential for color and expression. This chapter explores the beautiful world of fostering creativity in children with Down Syndrome. By providing opportunities for artistic exploration and communication, you can help your child tap into their unique voice and unleash their inner artist.

Why Artistic Expression Matters

Creativity is not just about creating beautiful things; it is about exploring, expressing emotions, and seeing the world in a new light. Here is why fostering creativity is important for children with Down Syndrome:

- **Boosts Self-Esteem:** Engaging in creative activities allows your child to experience a sense of accomplishment and pride in their creations.

- **Improves Communication:** Art can be a powerful tool for communication, especially for children who might struggle with verbal expression.

- **Cognitive Development:** Creative activities stimulate the brain, enhance problem-solving skills, and promote cognitive development.

- **Emotional Outlet:** Art provides a safe space for your child to express their emotions and explore their inner world.

Exploring Artistic Avenues

There are endless possibilities when it comes to fostering creativity. Here are some ideas to get you started:

- **Visual Arts:** Painting, drawing, sculpting, and collage are fantastic ways for your child to explore colors, textures, and shapes.

- **Music and Movement:** Singing, dancing, playing instruments, or creating their own rhythms can be a joyful and expressive experience.

- **Drama and Storytelling:** Encourage storytelling through role-playing, puppet shows, or creating mini-plays.

- **The Sensory World:** Activities that explore different textures, sounds, and smells can spark creativity and engage your child's senses.

Remember

- **Focus on the Process, Not the Product:** The most important thing is for your child to enjoy the experience of creating. Do not get hung up on the final outcome.

- **Celebrate Uniqueness:** Every child is unique, and their art will be too! Encourage your child to express themselves freely and celebrate their individual style.

- **Make it Fun and Accessible:** Keep activities fun and engaging. Use simple materials readily available at home. Adapt activities as needed to suit your child's abilities and interests.

Beyond the Chapter: A Journey of Self-Discovery and Expression

This chapter has opened the door to fostering creativity in your child. Remember, creativity is a journey of self-discovery and expression. By providing a nurturing environment filled with opportunities for exploration, you will be nurturing the artistic spark within your child. Watch as they blossom, expressing themselves through vibrant colors, captivating rhythms, and imaginative stories - a testament to their unique voice and inner world. You will be their biggest supporter, cheering them on as they unleash their creativity and paint their own masterpiece on the canvas of life.

17. DEVELOPING WORK SKILLS

Imagine your child as a budding seed, brimming with potential to grow strong and independent. This chapter explores the exciting world of vocational training, equipping your child with Down Syndrome with the skills they need to flourish in the workforce. By fostering independence and providing opportunities for meaningful work, you will be nurturing a future filled with purpose and accomplishment.

Why Work Matters: The Value of Employment

Employment is not just about earning money. It is about building confidence, developing self-esteem, and fostering a sense of accomplishment. Here is why work matters for children with Down Syndrome:

- **Independence and Empowerment:** Having a job empowers your child to become more independent and contribute to their community.

- **Socialization and Interaction:** The workplace provides opportunities for socialization and interaction with colleagues, fostering new friendships and building social skills.

- **Structure and Routine:** Employment brings structure and routine into your child's life, promoting a sense of purpose and responsibility.

- **Personal Growth:** Learning new skills on the job can boost confidence and self-esteem, paving the way for further personal growth.

Exploring Vocational Training Options

There are many paths to successful employment for children with Down Syndrome. Here is how to explore vocational training opportunities:

- **Early Identification of Interests:** Pay attention to your child's interests and talents. What activities do they enjoy? This can be a starting point for exploring career options.

- **School Programs:** Many schools offer vocational training programs that can equip your child with valuable job skills.

- **Community Resources:** Several community organizations and agencies specialize in vocational training for individuals with disabilities. Seek guidance from social workers or career counselors.

Essential Work Skills for Success

Here are some key work skills you can help your child develop:

- **Communication Skills:** Effective communication is crucial in any workplace. Help your child learn to ask for clarification, follow instructions, and communicate clearly.

- **Problem-Solving Skills:** Encourage your child to think independently and brainstorm solutions to small work-related challenges.

- **Time Management:** Developing good time management skills helps your child stay organized and complete tasks efficiently.

- **Social Skills:** Strong social skills enable your child to build rapport with colleagues and navigate workplace interactions.

- **Self-Advocacy:** Encourage your child to speak up for themselves and express their needs in a respectful and confident manner.

Remember

- **Start Early:** Begin thinking about vocational training early on. Expose your child to different work environments and activities to explore their interests.

- **Celebrate Milestones:** Acknowledge and celebrate your child's progress, no matter how small. Positive reinforcement keeps them motivated.

- **Focus on Abilities:** Focus on your child's strengths and abilities, not their limitations. Every person brings unique skills and talents to the workplace.

Beyond the Chapter: A Journey of Growth and Independence

This chapter has equipped you with knowledge and resources for fostering work skills in your child. Remember, vocational training is a journey of growth and independence. By providing support, exploring opportunities, and celebrating their achievements, you will be empowering your child to navigate the world of work with confidence. Watch them blossom, contributing their talents and skills to the world, painting their own unique masterpiece on the canvas of a fulfilling career. You will be their guide and cheerleader, supporting them every step of the way.

18. BUILDING HEALTHY RELATIONSHIPS

Imagine your child as a beautiful flower, yearning for connection and love. This chapter explores the delicate world of building healthy relationships for children with Down Syndrome. By providing open communication, guidance, and a foundation of love, you can help your child navigate the world of friendships, dating, and sexuality with confidence and respect.

Understanding Needs and Emotions: Recognizing the Desire for Connection

Just like everyone else, children with Down Syndrome have emotional needs and a desire for connection. Here is why communication is key:

- **Socialization is Essential:** Healthy relationships foster a sense of belonging, provide companionship, and teach valuable social skills.

- **Open Communication is Key:** Talking openly about relationships, dating, and sexuality allows you to address concerns and provide your child with accurate information.

- **Respecting Individuality:** Every child develops at their own pace. Respect your child's individual needs and preferences regarding relationships.

Building Blocks for Healthy Relationships

Here are some steps to foster healthy relationships in your child's life:

- **Start Early:** Conversations about friendship, communication, and respect can start young. Use age-appropriate language and build a foundation of understanding.

- **Social Skills Development:** Encourage opportunities for social interaction through group activities, clubs, or social skills groups.

- **Setting Boundaries:** Talk to your child about healthy boundaries in relationships, including respect for personal space and appropriate touch.

- **Body Positivity and Self-Esteem:** Promote a positive body image and healthy self-esteem in your child. This empowers them to build strong and healthy relationships.

- **Open Communication:** Create a safe space for your child to ask questions and express concerns about relationships, dating, and sexuality.

Understanding Sexuality

Talking about sexuality can feel awkward, but it is an important conversation to have with your child with Down Syndrome. Here are some tips for approaching the topic:

- **Age-Appropriate Information:** Provide information about sexuality that is appropriate for your child's age and understanding level.

- **Focus on Consent:** Emphasize the importance of consent in relationships. Teach your child that "no" means no, regardless of the situation.

- **Respecting Choices:** Respect your child's choices and preferences regarding relationships. Your role is to guide and support, not dictate their decisions.

Remember

- **Be Patient:** It takes time for children to develop social and emotional skills. Be patient and understanding as your child navigates the world of relationships.

- **Seek Professional Guidance:** Do not hesitate to seek guidance from therapists, social workers, or counselors who specialize in working with individuals with Down Syndrome.

- **Love and Support Above All:** Provide your child with unconditional love and support as they explore different aspects of relationships. Let them know you are always there to listen and guide them.

Beyond the Chapter: A Journey of Love, Growth, and Respect

This chapter has opened the door to fostering healthy relationships for your child. Remember, building healthy relationships is a journey of love, growth, and respect. By providing open communication, safe spaces for exploration, and unwavering support, you will be nurturing the garden of your child's emotional well-being. Watch them blossom with confidence as they build meaningful connections, discover their desires, and navigate the beautiful world of relationships. You will be their gardener, providing the love and sunlight they need to bloom and thrive.

19. COPING WITH GRIEF & LOSS

Life is a beautiful journey filled with love, laughter, and sometimes, loss. This chapter explores the difficult topic of grief and loss, specifically for families caring for a loved one with Down Syndrome. It offers guidance on supporting yourself and your loved one as you navigate this challenging time.

Understanding Grief

Grief is a natural response to loss. It is a wave of emotions that can feel overwhelming at times. Here is what to expect:

- **A Range of Emotions:** Grief can manifest in many ways, including sadness, anger, frustration, guilt, or even disbelief. It is important to acknowledge and accept all your emotions without judgment.

- **Individual Experiences:** Everyone grieves differently. Some people experience intense emotions immediately, while others might grieve more gradually. There is no right or wrong way to grieve.

- **Allowing Time:** Healing takes time. Be patient with yourself and your loved one as you navigate the journey of grief.

Taking Care of Your Well-Being

While caring for your loved one, it is crucial to take care of your own well-being. Here are some ways to do that:

- **Seek Support:** Do not bottle up your emotions. Talk to a trusted friend, family member, therapist, or a support group for parents of children with Down Syndrome.

- **Maintain Healthy Habits:** Prioritize healthy habits like eating nutritious meals, getting enough sleep, and exercising regularly. These practices build resilience and help you manage stress.

- **Allow Time for Self-Care:** Schedule activities you enjoy, even if it is just taking a relaxing bath or reading a book. Taking care of yourself allows you to better care for your loved one.

Supporting Your Loved One with Down Syndrome: Understanding and Communication

People with Down Syndrome experience grief differently. Here are some ways to support your loved one:

- **Open Communication:** Maintain open and honest communication. Use simple language and explain the loss in a way that is easy for them to understand.

- **Maintain Routines:** Maintaining familiar routines provides comfort and stability during a time of change. However, be flexible and adjust routines as needed.

- **Visual Aids:** Visual aids like pictures or memory boxes can help your loved one process their emotions and remember the person they lost.

- **Be Patient:** It might take your loved one longer to understand the concept of death. Be patient and offer reassurance.

A Path to Healing

There are resources available to help you and your loved one cope with grief. Here are some to explore:

- **Support Groups:** Connecting with other families who have experienced loss can be incredibly helpful. Share experiences, offer and receive support, and learn coping strategies together.

- **Grief Counseling:** Consider seeking professional grief counseling for yourself or your loved one. A therapist can provide guidance and support during this difficult time.

Remember

- **Grief is a Process:** There is no linear path to healing. Allow yourself and your loved one to grieve in your own way and at your own pace.

- **Celebrate Memories:** It is okay to smile and share happy memories of the person you lost. Celebrating their life alongside grieving their absence is a healthy part of the process.

- **Seek Help if Needed:** Do not hesitate to seek professional help if you or your loved one are struggling to cope with grief.

Beyond the Chapter: A Journey of Love and Resilience

This chapter has equipped you with tools and

resources to navigate grief and loss. Remember, grief is a journey, not a destination. By supporting yourself, your loved one, and seeking help when needed, you can find strength and resilience to move forward together. The love shared with your loved one with Down syndrome creates a bond that endures, even in the face of loss.

20. LEARNING AND GROWING FROM YOUR CHILD'S JOURNEY

Imagine your child as a sparkling diamond, each facet reflecting unique beauty and strength. This chapter explores the transformative journey of raising a child with Down syndrome. By embracing the challenges and celebrating the triumphs with love, you will discover a world of personal growth, acceptance, and deeper appreciation for life.

Learning to See the World Through New Eyes: Embracing a Different Path

Parenting a child with Down syndrome can be an unexpected journey. Here is why embracing a different perspective is key:

- **Shifting Expectations:** Letting go of preconceived notions and embracing your child's unique abilities opens doors to a world of joy and wonder.

- **Celebrating Milestones:** Each victory, no matter how small, is a cause for celebration. Redefining success through your child's eyes fosters a deeper connection.

- **Appreciating the Simple Joys:** Children with Down syndrome often possess a pure joy for life and a keen appreciation for simple things. Their perspective reminds us to savor the beauty in everyday moments.

Growing Together: A Journey of Discovery and Strength

Raising a child with Down syndrome can be a catalyst for personal growth. Here is how:

- **Developing Patience and Resilience:** Navigating challenges and advocating for your child's needs strengthens your patience and resilience.

- **Discovering New Strengths:** You will discover hidden strengths and a newfound determination to support your child's dreams and aspirations.

- **Building a Strong Support Network:** Connecting with other families and caregivers fosters a sense of community and shared understanding.

The Gift of Love: Fueling Growth and Embracing the Journey

Love is the cornerstone of any healthy parent-child relationship, and it is even more crucial when raising a child with Down syndrome. Here is why love matters:

- **Unconditional Acceptance:** Loving your child unconditionally fosters security and a strong sense of self-worth.

- **Celebrating Individuality:** Every child is unique, and your child with Down syndrome is no exception. Celebrate their individuality and embrace their special gifts.

- **Finding Joy in the Everyday:** Focus on the moments of laughter, joy, and connection. These are the treasures that enrich your life and your child's.

Remember

- **Every Family's Journey is Unique:** Do not compare your experience to others. Embrace your child's individual journey and create memories that will last a lifetime.

- **Focus on the Positive:** There will be challenges, but choose to focus on the positive aspects of parenting your child. Find joy in their laughter, celebrate their successes, and cherish the special bond you share.

- **Advocate for Your Child:** Be your child's voice and advocate for their needs. Educate yourself and others about Down syndrome and create a world of acceptance and inclusion.

Beyond the Chapter: A Lifetime of Love and Learning

This chapter has reminded you of the transformative power of raising a child with Down syndrome. The journey may not be what you expected, but it is a journey filled with love, learning, and growth. Embrace the unexpected, celebrate your child's unique gifts, and hold onto the joy of watching them blossom. You will discover that the greatest gift of all is the love you share and the beautiful lessons learned along the way. You are not just raising a child; you are learning to see the world through a lens of love, acceptance, and unwavering appreciation for life.

21. LEAVING A LEGACY

Imagine your child as a pebble, tossed into a still pond. Their journey with Down syndrome creates ripples that can touch countless lives. This chapter explores the power of leaving a legacy – a legacy built on love, advocacy, and sharing your story. By educating others, raising awareness, and inspiring positive change, you can create a lasting impact that extends far beyond your family.

The Ripple Effect: Sharing Your Experiences for Positive Change

Your journey as a parent of a child with Down syndrome holds valuable lessons and insights. Here is how sharing your story can create a ripple effect:

- **Breaking Down Barriers:** Sharing your experiences can help break down stereotypes and misconceptions about Down syndrome.

- **Promoting Inclusion:** By educating others about your child's abilities, you can advocate for a more inclusive world where everyone can thrive.

- **Inspiring Others:** Your story can be a source of strength and encouragement for other families navigating similar journeys.

Spreading Awareness Through Different Avenues

There are many ways to share your story and leave a positive legacy:

- **Talking Openly:** Start by talking openly about your child and Down syndrome with friends, family, and your community. Open conversations foster empathy and understanding.

- **Sharing on Social Media:** Use social media platforms to showcase your child's abilities and experiences. Share positive stories and raise awareness about Down syndrome.

- **Advocacy Groups:** Connect with advocacy groups dedicated to Down syndrome. Get involved in awareness campaigns, fundraising events, or volunteer your time.

- **Creating Resources:** Consider writing a blog, creating a website, or even a children's book that shares your experiences and educates others about Down syndrome.

Remember

- **Start Small, Dream Big:** You do not have to change the world overnight. Start by making small changes in your own community and let your impact grow organically.

- **Focus on the Positive:** Share your story with a positive and hopeful perspective. Highlight your child's strengths and achievements.

- **Empowering Your Child:** As your child grows older, involve them in sharing their story too. Empower them to advocate for themselves and inspire others.

Beyond the Chapter: A Journey of Love and Impact

This chapter has empowered you to leave a lasting legacy. Your journey with your child is an opportunity to create positive change in the world. By sharing your story, raising awareness, and advocating for inclusion, you can create a ripple effect of love and acceptance that extends far beyond your family. You will be leaving a legacy not just for your child, but for generations to come. Your love, your strength, and your courage will pave the way for a more inclusive and understanding world.

22. TECHNOLOGY & DOWN SYNDROME

Imagine your child as a curious explorer, eager to discover the world. This chapter explores the exciting world of technology and how it can empower your child with Down syndrome. By utilizing assistive tools for learning and communication, you can unlock their potential and help them navigate the world with confidence and independence.

Technology for Bridging Gaps and Fostering Learning

Technology is not just for entertainment; it can be a powerful tool for learning and communication. Here is why technology matters for children with Down syndrome:

- **Engaging Learning Experiences:** Technology offers interactive and engaging learning experiences that cater to different learning styles.

- **Personalized Learning:** Many apps and programs can be customized to meet your child's individual needs and learning pace.

- **Improved Communication Skills:** Communication apps and tools can help children who struggle with verbal communication express themselves more effectively.

- **Building Independence:** Assistive technology can empower your child to complete tasks independently, fostering a sense of accomplishment and self-esteem.

Exploring the Tech Tools for Every Need

There are many different types of assistive technology available, each with its own unique benefits. Here is a glimpse into the tech toolbox:

- **Educational Apps:** Look for apps that focus on specific learning goals like reading, math, vocabulary development, or social skills. Many apps incorporate interactive elements, games, and rewards to keep learning fun and engaging.

- **Augmentative and Alternative Communication (AAC) Tools:** These tools can help children who have difficulty speaking or using traditional communication methods. AAC tools may include picture boards, specialized tablets with voice output, or speech-generating software.

- **Accessibility Features:** Most smartphones and tablets come with built-in accessibility features like text-to-speech, screen magnification, and voice control. These features can make interacting with technology easier for children with visual or motor impairments.

- **Assistive Devices:** There are specialized devices available to assist with tasks like handwriting, organization, or learning time management.

Remember

- **Start Early:** Introduce technology early on to familiarize your child with its potential.

- **Choose the Right Tools:** Not all technology is created equal. Consider your child's needs, interests, and learning style when choosing apps and programs.

- **Supervision and Guidance:** While technology can be beneficial, it is important to provide supervision and guidance to ensure safe and responsible use. Set screen time limits and encourage other forms of play and learning.

Beyond the Chapter: A Journey of Discovery and

Independence

This chapter has opened the door to the exciting world of technology for children with Down syndrome. Remember, technology is a powerful tool to enhance learning, communication, and independence. By exploring different tools, finding the right fit for your child, and providing support and guidance, you can equip them to navigate the digital world with confidence. Watch them explore, learn, and connect with the world around them through the magic of technology. You will be their guide, helping them unlock their potential and embrace a future filled with possibilities.

23. BUILDING A DIVERSE & INCLUSIVE COMMUNITY

Imagine your child as a vibrant flower in a beautiful garden. This chapter explores the importance of building a diverse and inclusive community, a garden where all flowers can blossom and thrive. By fostering acceptance with love, you can create a world where your child with Down syndrome feels valued, respected, and celebrated for their unique individuality.

The Power of Belonging

A strong and inclusive community provides your child with a sense of belonging, acceptance, and connection. Here is why it matters:

- **Social Interaction and Friendship:** Being part of a diverse community allows your child to build friendships, develop social skills, and feel a sense of belonging.

- **Acceptance and Understanding:** In an inclusive environment, your child feels valued for who they are, fostering confidence and self-esteem.

- **Learning and Growth:** Interacting with people from different backgrounds can broaden your child's perspective and understanding of the world.

Planting Seeds of Acceptance

Here are some ways to cultivate a more inclusive and accepting community for your child:

- **Open Communication:** Talk openly with your family, friends, and neighbors about Down syndrome. Educate them about your child's abilities and dispel any misconceptions.

- **Inclusive Activities:** Seek out opportunities for your child to participate in activities with typically developing peers. This could be anything from sports teams and clubs to after-school programs.

- **Advocacy in Action:** Speak up for your child and advocate for their inclusion in different settings. Talk to school administrators, community center leaders, or park officials about creating more inclusive environments.

- **Celebrating Differences:** Help others celebrate the unique qualities and abilities of your child with Down syndrome. Everyone has something special to offer, and diversity enriches all our lives.

Remember

- **Lead by Example:** Be a role model for acceptance and inclusion. Treat everyone with kindness and respect, and encourage your child to do the same.

- **Patience and Persistence:** Building an inclusive community takes time and effort. Be patient and persistent in your efforts to create a world where everyone feels welcome and valued.

- **Celebrate Milestones:** Celebrate moments of acceptance and inclusion, no matter how small. Positive reinforcement encourages others to continue fostering a welcoming environment.

Beyond the Chapter: A Journey of Growth Together

This chapter has empowered you to build a more inclusive community. Remember, fostering acceptance is not just about creating a better world for your child; it is about creating a better world for everyone. By working together, celebrating diversity, and leading by example, you can nurture a garden of acceptance where all flowers, including your child, can bloom with confidence and joy. You will be nurturing not just your child, but the entire community, creating a world where everyone feels seen, heard, and valued for who they are.

24. FAITH & SPIRITUALITY

Imagine your child as a tiny sailboat navigating a vast ocean. This chapter explores the calming power of faith and spirituality, a guiding light that can offer comfort, strength, and hope on the journey of raising a child with Down syndrome. By nurturing your own beliefs and sharing them with your child in a loving and respectful way, you can create a sense of peace and purpose for your entire family.

Finding Solace in Belief: Why Faith Matters

Faith and spirituality can provide a sense of comfort, strength, and meaning during challenging times. Here is why it can be valuable for families with Down syndrome:

- **Inner Strength:** Faith can be a source of strength, helping you navigate difficult emotions and find peace amidst uncertainty.

- **Community and Support:** Religious communities often offer emotional support and a sense of belonging, connecting you with others facing similar challenges.

- **Finding Purpose:** Faith can help you find purpose in your journey, reminding you that your child's life has meaning and value.

Nurturing Your Beliefs

There are many different paths to faith and spirituality. Here are some ways to nurture your beliefs:

- **Prayer or Meditation:** Dedicate time for prayer or meditation, seeking guidance, expressing gratitude, and finding inner peace.

- **Religious Services:** Attend religious services if they align with your beliefs. They can provide a sense of community and spiritual nourishment.

- **Gratitude Practice:** Focus on the positive aspects of your life with your child. Practice gratitude for their unique gifts and the joy they bring.

Sharing Faith with Your Child: A Journey of Exploration

Children with Down syndrome can experience and connect with faith in unique ways. Here is how to share your beliefs with your child:

- **Simple Teachings:** Start with simple teachings about your faith, focusing on concepts like love, compassion, and helping others.
- **Rituals and Traditions:** If your faith involves rituals or traditions, incorporate them in a way your child can understand and participate in.

- **Focus on Meaning:** Help your child connect your faith to their own lives. Discuss how your beliefs guide your actions and inspire you to be kind and loving.

Remember

- **Respect Individual Beliefs:** Respect your child's individual beliefs and preferences as they grow older. Faith is a personal journey for everyone.

- **Find What Works for You:** There is no right or wrong way to practice faith. Find what brings you and your family comfort and meaning.

- **Focus on Love:** Above all, remember that love is the foundation of everything. Let your love be the guiding light as you navigate your faith journey with your child.

Beyond the Chapter: A Journey of Hope and Strength

This chapter has reminded you of the power of faith and spirituality. Whether you find solace in a specific religion or connect with a higher power in your own way, faith can be a source of strength, comfort, and hope. By nurturing your own beliefs and sharing them with your child in a loving and respectful way, you will be creating a guiding light for your family on the beautiful journey of raising a child with Down syndrome. Together, you will navigate the waves of life with faith as your anchor and love as your compass.

25. TRAVEL & ADVENTURE

Imagine your child as a curious explorer, yearning to discover the world. This chapter explores the exciting world of travel and adventure, creating unforgettable experiences that strengthen your bond and create lasting memories for your entire family. By planning trips that cater to your child's needs and interests, you can embark on a journey of exploration, laughter, and learning together.

The World Awaits: Why Travel Matters

Traveling with a child with Down syndrome can be enriching and rewarding for everyone involved. Here is why travel matters:

- **Creating Memories:** Traveling creates unique and unforgettable memories that you and your child will cherish forever.

- **Bonding Experiences:** Exploring new places together strengthens your family bond and fosters a sense of shared adventure.

- **Building Confidence:** Navigating new places and experiences can boost your child's confidence and sense of independence.

- **Exposure to Diversity:** Travel broadens your child's perspective and allows them to experience different cultures and ways of life.

Planning Your Adventure

Planning is key to a successful and enjoyable travel experience with your child. Here are some tips to consider:

- **Choose Your Destination Wisely:** Select a location that caters to your child's interests and abilities. Research accessibility options and choose destinations with child-friendly activities.

- **Plan Activities:** Plan activities that your child will enjoy, like visiting museums, exploring nature parks, or participating in local cultural events. Consider incorporating activities that stimulate their senses and encourage interaction with new environments.

- **Pack Smart:** Pack familiar items that bring comfort to your child, such as favorite toys, blankets, or sensory items. Be sure to pack all necessary medications and any adaptive equipment your child might need.

- **Prepare for Sensory Overload:** Travel can be overwhelming for some children. Plan for breaks, incorporate calming activities, and choose environments that cater to your child's sensory sensitivities.

- **Embrace Flexibility:** Be prepared to adjust your plans or itinerary based on your child's needs. Focus on creating fun and positive experiences rather than sticking to a rigid schedule.

Making Memories Together: Let the Adventure Begin!

Here are some ideas to inspire your travel adventures:

- **Family Getaways:** Plan a weekend getaway to a nearby beach resort, a charming mountain town, or a historical city with child-friendly attractions.

- **Educational Adventures:** Visit museums with interactive exhibits, historical sites, or natural wonders like national parks or zoos. These experiences can spark curiosity and create opportunities for learning.

- **Cultural Exploration:** Immerse yourselves in a different culture by exploring local markets, trying new foods, or attending traditional festivals. These experiences can broaden your child's perspective and foster appreciation for diversity.

Remember

- **Focus on Your Child:** Plan your trip around your child's interests and abilities. Choose destinations and activities that will create a positive and enjoyable experience for them.

- **Safety First:** Always prioritize your child's safety. Research the destination's medical facilities and accessibility options.

- **Celebrate Every Milestone:** Celebrate small victories, like navigating unfamiliar environments or trying new things. Positive reinforcement builds confidence and encourages further exploration.

Beyond the Chapter: A Lifetime of Exploration

This chapter has opened the door to the exciting world of travel with your child with Down syndrome. Remember, travel is not just about the destination; it is about the journey itself. By planning thoughtful adventures, embracing flexibility, and focusing on creating positive experiences, you will be creating a lifetime of memories and fostering a love for exploration for your entire family. The world awaits, filled with countless adventures to discover together. So pack your bags, unleash your sense of adventure, and embark on a journey of laughter, learning, and lasting memories with your child.

26. SIBLING SUPPORT GROUPS

Imagine your family as a beautiful tree, with each branch supporting the others. This chapter explores the importance of sibling support groups. Just like strong branches support the entire tree, sibling support groups provide a safe space for brothers and sisters of children with Down syndrome to connect, share experiences, and build a network of understanding.

Why Siblings Matter: Understanding Their Unique Journey

Having a sibling with Down syndrome can be an enriching experience, but it can also come with challenges. Here is why sibling support groups are valuable:

- **Unique Challenges:** Siblings may experience feelings of isolation, jealousy, or worry about their brother or sister with Down syndrome. Support groups allow them to share these feelings openly with others who understand.

- **Building Confidence:** Connecting with other siblings who share similar experiences can boost confidence and a sense of belonging.

- **Learning and Sharing:** Support groups provide a platform to learn coping mechanisms, communication strategies, and tips for navigating family dynamics.

Exploring Sibling Support Groups

There are many different types of sibling support groups available. Here is how to find the right fit:

- **Ask Your Doctor:** Talk to your child's doctor or therapist about local sibling support groups.

- **Online Resources:** Search online for national organizations dedicated to Down syndrome that offer sibling support programs or resources.

- **School Counselors:** Connect with your school counselor who might be aware of local support groups for siblings.

What to Expect in a Support Group:

Sibling support groups are typically facilitated by professionals or experienced parents. Here is what you might experience:

- **Open Discussions:** These groups offer a safe space for siblings to share their experiences, feelings, and concerns about having a brother or sister with Down syndrome.

- **Activities and Games:** Support groups may incorporate games, activities, or creative exercises to help siblings express themselves and learn new coping mechanisms.

- **Guest Speakers:** Sometimes, professionals like therapists or educators may be invited to speak on topics relevant to siblings of children with Down syndrome.

Remember

- **Not Everyone Needs a Group:** Some siblings may not feel comfortable participating in a group setting. Respect your child's decision and explore alternative forms of support.

- **Open Communication at Home:** Even if your child participates in a support group, maintain open communication at home. Create a safe space for them to share their feelings and experiences with you.

- **Celebrate Each Other:** Acknowledge and celebrate the unique bond between your children. Siblings play a vital role in each other's lives, offering love, support, and a lifelong connection.

Beyond the Chapter: A Strong and Supportive Family Tree

This chapter has highlighted the importance of sibling support groups. Remember, just like each branch strengthens the entire tree, sibling support groups offer a strong network for brothers and sisters of children with Down syndrome. By connecting with others who understand, sharing experiences, and learning valuable coping mechanisms, siblings can build confidence, navigate challenges, and thrive within their unique family dynamic. With open communication, encouragement, and the support of sibling connections, your family tree will continue to grow strong and resilient.

27. CARING FOR YOURSELF AS A CARE GIVER

Imagine yourself as a loving gardener, tending to a beautiful flower – your child with Down syndrome. This chapter explores the importance of self-care for caregivers. Just like a gardener needs to tend to their own needs to nurture the flowers, you need to care for yourself to have the energy and love to support your child. By prioritizing your well-being, you will be better equipped to create a joyful and fulfilling life for your entire family.

Why Self-Care Matters

Taking care of yourself is not selfish; it is essential. Here is why self-care matters for caregivers of children with Down syndrome:

- **Preventing Burnout:** The constant demands of caregiving can lead to exhaustion and burnout. Self-care helps you recharge and maintain your emotional and physical well-being.

- **Enhanced Patience and Positivity:** When you are well-rested and feel good, you will have more patience and a positive attitude to navigate challenges with your child.

- **Stronger Bond with Your Child:** By taking care of yourself, you will be more present and emotionally available to connect and enjoy moments with your child.

Simple Strategies for Self-Care

Self-care does not have to be complicated or expensive. Here are some simple strategies to incorporate into your routine:

- **Schedule Time for Yourself:** Even if it is just 30 minutes a day, dedicate time for activities you enjoy, like reading, taking a relaxing bath, or spending time in nature.

- **Connect with Others:** Nurture your relationships with friends and family. Talk to someone you trust about your challenges and joys as a caregiver.

- **Seek Support:** Do not be afraid to ask for help from your partner, family members, or friends. Consider respite care options that allow you to take a break from caregiving duties.

- **Physical Activity:** Engage in regular physical activity, even if it is just a brisk walk or some gentle yoga. Exercise releases endorphins, which can improve mood and reduce stress.

- **Healthy Habits:** Prioritize good sleep, healthy eating habits, and relaxation techniques like meditation or deep breathing exercises to manage stress.

Remember

- **Self-Care is Not Selfish:** Taking care of yourself is not a luxury; it is a necessity. A well-rested and healthy caregiver is better equipped to provide loving and consistent care for their child.

- **Start Small:** Do not overwhelm yourself. Begin with small, manageable self-care practices and gradually build them into your routine.

- **Seek Support Groups:** Connect with other caregivers who understand your unique challenges. Sharing experiences and learning coping strategies can be a source of strength and encouragement.

Beyond the Chapter: A Journey of Love and Growth

This chapter has empowered you to prioritize your

well-being. Remember, caring for your child with Down syndrome is a lifelong journey filled with love, challenges, and growth. By taking care of yourself, you will be pouring love and energy back into your own cup, allowing you to overflow with love and dedication for your child. You are not just a caregiver; you are the foundation of your family's well-being. By nurturing yourself, you will create a strong and loving environment where everyone can thrive.

28. LEGAL ADVOCACY

Imagine your child as a superhero, with incredible potential waiting to be unleashed. This chapter explores the world of legal advocacy – your role as a champion for your child's rights. By understanding the law and advocating for your child's needs, you can help them reach their full potential and live a fulfilling life.

Knowing Your Rights: A Foundation for Advocacy

Everyone, including individuals with Down syndrome, has basic rights. Here is why understanding the law is crucial:

- **Equal Opportunities:** Laws ensure equal access to education, healthcare, employment, and other important aspects of life.

- **Protection from Discrimination:** It is illegal to discriminate against someone based on their disability. Knowing your rights empowers you to fight for fair treatment.

- **Making Informed Decisions:** Understanding legal options allows you to make informed decisions about your child's education, healthcare, and future.

Becoming Your Child's Champion: Steps to Effective Advocacy

Advocacy is not about being a lawyer; it is about being your child's voice. Here are some ways to become an effective advocate:

- **Educate Yourself:** Learn about the laws that protect individuals with Down syndrome, including education rights, healthcare benefits, and employment opportunities.

- **Connect with Advocacy Groups:** National and local Down syndrome organizations offer resources, support, and guidance on advocating for your child's rights.

- **Communicate Openly:** Maintain open communication with your child's doctor, teachers, and other service providers. Clearly articulate your child's needs and advocate for appropriate accommodations.

- **Know Your Rights, Raise Your Voice:** If you encounter discrimination or feel your child's rights are being violated, do not be afraid to speak up. Seek legal guidance if necessary.

Remember

- **You Are Not Alone:** Many parents and families advocate for the rights of individuals with Down syndrome. Connect with them for support and encouragement.

- **Start Small, Stay Consistent:** Advocacy can be a long-term process. Start small, like advocating for an Individualized Education Program (IEP) at school, and be persistent in your efforts.

- **Focus on Positive Change:** Approach advocacy with a positive and solution-oriented mindset. Focus on creating a more inclusive and supportive environment for your child and others with Down syndrome.

Beyond the Chapter: A Legacy of Empowerment

This chapter has ignited your passion for legal advocacy. Remember, by standing up for your child's rights, you are not just fighting for them; you are fighting for a brighter future for all individuals with Down syndrome. Your advocacy has the power to break down barriers, ensure equal opportunities, and empower your child to reach their full potential. You are your child's hero, championing their rights and paving the way for a more inclusive world.

29. SEXUALITY EDUCATION

Imagine your child as a budding flower, blossoming into a young adult. This chapter explores the importance of sexuality education for children with Down syndrome. Just like nurturing a flower requires the right care, providing open and honest communication about sexuality equips your child to navigate their feelings, develop healthy relationships, and understand their body.

Why Sexuality Education Matters

Many parents may hesitate to discuss sexuality with their child with Down syndrome. However, sexuality education is crucial for several reasons:

- **Building Confidence and Self-Esteem:** Understanding their bodies and sexuality empowers your child and promotes a healthy sense of self.

- **Developing Healthy Relationships:** Sexuality education can help your child develop appropriate boundaries, identify healthy relationships, and avoid potential exploitation.

- **Safety and Risk Awareness:** Education can teach your child to recognize and avoid risky situations, as well as how to report inappropriate behavior.

How to Approach Sexuality Education

Sexuality education should be an ongoing conversation, not a one-time talk. Here is how to approach this topic with love and understanding:

- **Start Early:** Simple conversations about body parts, privacy, and appropriate touch can begin early on and gradually become more detailed as your child grows older.

- **Use Clear and Simple Language:** Avoid using confusing jargon or euphemisms. Focus on using correct anatomical terms and explain concepts in a way your child can understand.

- **Be Open and Honest:** Create a safe space for your child to ask questions without judgment. Be prepared to answer their questions honestly and directly.

- **Respect Their Privacy:** As your child matures, respect their developing sense of privacy. Offer support and guidance, but avoid intruding on their personal life.

Setting Boundaries and Fostering Healthy Relationships

Sexuality education goes beyond just body parts. Here are some additional aspects to consider:

- **Healthy Touch and Boundaries:** Teach your child about consent and the importance of respecting other people's physical boundaries.

- **Identifying Abuse:** Explain what inappropriate touching or behavior looks like and empower your child to speak up if they feel uncomfortable.

- **Social Skills and Relationships:** Help your child develop social skills and navigate different types of relationships, from friendships to romantic connections.

Remember

- **Tailor It to Your Child:** Every child learns and develops at their own pace. Adapt your approach based on your child's individual needs and understanding.

- **Seek Professional Guidance:** If you feel overwhelmed, do not hesitate to seek professional guidance from therapists, social workers, or organizations experienced in sexuality education for individuals with Down syndrome.

- **Open Communication is Key:** Maintain open and ongoing communication with your child. Let them know you are always available to answer their questions and address their concerns.

Beyond the Chapter: A Journey of Growth and Love

This chapter has empowered you to navigate sexuality education with confidence. Remember, your role is to guide your child with love, respect, and open communication. By creating a safe and supportive environment, you will equip them with the knowledge and skills they need to blossom into a confident and healthy young adult. Together, you can navigate this journey and foster healthy relationships, safety, and understanding in your child's life.

30. END-OF-LIFE CARE

Imagine your child as a beautiful sunset, painting the sky with vibrant colors before gently fading away. This chapter explores the sensitive topic of end-of-life care for individuals with Down syndrome. By planning ahead with love and compassion, you can ensure your child receives dignified and comfortable care during their final days, while cherishing the precious moments you have together.

Facing the Future with Love: Why End-of-Life Care Matters

While no one wants to think about losing a loved one, planning for end-of-life care is an act of love. Here is why it is important:

- **Honoring Your Child's Wishes:** By discussing and documenting your child's preferences for care, you ensure their wishes are respected during their final days.

- **Alleviating Stress:** Planning ahead reduces stress and confusion for you and other family members during a difficult time.

- **Making Informed Decisions:** Open communication and planning allow everyone involved to make informed decisions about your child's care.

Planning for a Peaceful Journey

End-of-life care planning focuses on your child's comfort, dignity, and your family's emotional well-being. Here are some key steps:

- **Start Early Conversations:** While still young, initiate open conversations with your child about their hopes and fears regarding end-of-life care, adapting the discussion as they mature.

- **Choose a Healthcare Proxy:** Appoint a trusted individual to make medical decisions on your child's behalf if they are unable to speak for themselves.

- **Create an Advance Directive:** This legal document outlines your child's wishes for medical treatment, pain management, and end-of-life care preferences.

- **Consider Hospice Care:** Hospice care focuses on comfort and quality of life for terminally ill patients. Explore hospice options that cater to the specific needs of individuals with Down syndrome.

- **Talk to Your Loved Ones:** Involve close family members and caregivers in your discussions and planning to ensure everyone is aware of your child's wishes.

Remember

- **Focus on Comfort and Respect:** The goal of end-of-life care is to ensure your child's comfort, dignity, and pain management during their final days.

- **Seek Support:** Dealing with end-of-life care can be emotionally challenging. Do not hesitate to seek support from therapists, counselors, or spiritual advisors.

- **Cherish Every Moment:** As you plan for the future, cherish the present. Create lasting memories and celebrate the life and love you share with your child.

Beyond the Chapter: A Journey of Love and Acceptance

This chapter has opened a dialogue about the sensitive but essential topic of end-of-life care. Remember, planning for this difficult time is an act of profound love. By making informed decisions and cherishing every moment, you can ensure your child receives the care they deserve during their final stages, while navigating this journey with acceptance and love. The memories you create together will continue to shine brightly long after the sunset.

31. A DAY IN OUR LIVES

Imagine a vibrant tapestry, woven with threads of love, laughter, frustration, and accomplishment. This chapter offers a glimpse into a typical day in the life of a family with a child with Down syndrome. Just like every tapestry is unique, every family's journey is different. This chapter celebrates the love that binds you together, acknowledges the challenges you may face, and highlights the triumphs, big and small, that make your family extraordinary.

A Blend of Routine and Surprise

The day begins like many others, with the gentle hum of morning routines. Your child might wake you up with a big smile and an enthusiastic greeting. Perhaps getting dressed takes a little longer, requiring patience and understanding. Breakfast might be a joyous celebration of favorite foods, or a negotiation to encourage a balanced meal. Each morning brings its own unique melody, a beautiful blend of routine and surprise.

Embracing Learning

For many children with Down syndrome, school is a bustling hub of learning and social interaction. Therapists might visit your home, helping your child develop new skills in speech, physical coordination, or social interaction. Afternoons might be filled with extracurricular activities, like swimming lessons, music classes, or playtime with friends. Every day is an opportunity for your child to learn, grow, and explore the world around them.

Challenges and Frustrations

Every family faces challenges. There might be moments of frustration when communication feels difficult, or a meltdown disrupts the evening routine. Perhaps doctor appointments or therapy sessions feel overwhelming. These challenges are a natural part of the journey, and it is important to acknowledge them. Remember, you are not alone. There are resources and support systems available to help you navigate these moments with compassion and understanding.

Celebrating Victories Big and Small

The true magic of this journey lies in celebrating victories, big and small. Maybe your child masters a new skill, says their first complete sentence, or makes a new friend. Perhaps they participate in a school play or proudly share their artwork. These moments are the sweet melodies that fill your life with joy and pride. Savor these triumphs, no matter how small they may seem. They are a testament to your child's hard work and your unwavering love and support.

The Evening Encore

As the day draws to a close, there is quiet time for snuggles, stories, and sharing the day's experiences. This is a time to reflect on the tapestry you are weaving together. There will be threads of laughter, tears, frustration, and accomplishment. But most importantly, there will be a vibrant thread of love, binding your family together.

Remember

- **Every Family's Tapestry is Unique:** There is no right or wrong way to navigate this journey. Embrace your family's individuality and celebrate the love that makes you strong.

- **Focus on the Positive:** While challenges are inevitable, focus on celebrating your child's victories and the joy they bring into your life.

- **Seek Support:** Do not hesitate to seek support from your partner, family, friends, and professional resources. You are not alone on this journey.

Beyond the Chapter: A Journey of Unconditional Love

This chapter has offered a glimpse into the beautiful

and complex world of raising a child with Down syndrome. Remember, this is a lifelong journey filled with love, laughter, challenges, and triumphs. Embrace the journey, celebrate the small victories, and cherish the love that binds your family together. Your tapestry of love and dedication will continue to grow and inspire others as you navigate this extraordinary adventure.

32. THE LANGUAGE OF LOVE

Imagine your child as a beautiful flower, needing sunshine and water to thrive. This chapter explores the concept of love languages – different ways people feel loved. Just like some flowers bloom best in bright sunlight, others flourish with gentle rain. By understanding your child's unique love language, you can express your affection in ways that truly resonate with them, nurturing their hearts and strengthening your bond.

Why Love Languages Matter

Everyone, including children with Down syndrome, has a primary love language – the way they feel most loved and appreciated. Here is why understanding love languages is important:

- **Stronger Bond and Deeper Connection:** Speaking your child's love language fosters a deeper connection and strengthens your emotional bond.

- **Enhanced Self-Esteem:** Feeling loved and appreciated boosts your child's confidence and self-esteem.

- **Improved Communication:** Understanding their love language allows you to communicate your love more effectively.

Discovering Your Child's Language: Unveiling the Clues

There are five main love languages: Words of affirmation, quality time, physical touch, acts of service, and gifts. Here are some tips to discover your child's primary language:

- **Observe Their Behavior:** Pay attention to how your child expresses love to others. Do they say "I love you" often, or do they prefer spending quality time together?

- **Listen to Their Requests:** Notice what your child asks for most often. Do they crave cuddles, or do they light up when you play a game together?

- **Consider Their Personality:** Some children are naturally affectionate, while others may prefer quiet moments of connection.

Speaking Their Language: Love in Action

Now that you have some clues, here are ways to

express love in each language:

- **Words of Affirmation:** Tell your child how much you love them, appreciate their efforts, and celebrate their achievements. Use descriptive words and sincere compliments.

- **Quality Time:** Put away distractions and focus on spending quality time with your child. Engage in activities they enjoy, listen attentively, and create special memories together.

- **Physical Touch:** Hugs, high fives, back rubs, and gentle cuddles can communicate love and affection. Respect your child's comfort level and tailor your approach to their needs.

- **Acts of Service:** Do helpful things for your child without being asked. Pack their favorite lunch, help them with a task they find challenging, or prepare their favorite snack.

- **Gifts:** While not the most important language, small gifts can be a way to show you are thinking of them. Focus on meaningful gestures like a favorite book, a handmade card, or tickets to a special event.

Remember

- **Love is a Combination:** Many children respond to a combination of love languages. Incorporate elements from each language to create a well-rounded expression of your love.

- **Be Flexible and Adaptable:** Your child's love language might change over time. Be observant and adapt your approach as needed.

- **The Most Important Language: Unconditional Love:** Above all, let your child know you love them unconditionally, no matter what. This is the foundation for a strong and healthy parent-child relationship.

Beyond the Chapter: A Lifetime of Love

This chapter has empowered you to speak your child's unique love language. Remember, by understanding how your child feels most loved, you can unlock the door to their heart and build a lifetime of connection. Your love and affection will nurture their spirit and help them blossom into a confident and happy individual.

33. LAUGHTER IS THE BEST MEDICINE

Imagine your family as a vibrant circus tent, filled with unexpected surprises and joyful moments. This chapter explores the power of laughter on your journey with Down syndrome. Just like a circus act can turn frowns upside down, humor can lighten the load, strengthen your bond, and create lasting memories. By embracing the funny moments and finding joy in the unexpected, you can turn your everyday experiences into a heartwarming and hilarious adventure.

Why Laughter Matters: The Magic Potion of Joy

Laughter is not just fun; it has real benefits for families with Down syndrome. Here is why laughter matters:

- **Stress Relief:** A good laugh can help reduce stress and anxiety, which can be common for both parents and children.

- **Stronger Bond:** Shared laughter creates positive memories and strengthens the emotional connection between you and your child.

- **Building Confidence:** Humor can help your child feel accepted and comfortable expressing themselves.

Uncovering the Laughter in Everyday Moments

Humor can be found in the most unexpected places. Here are some ways to embrace the funny on your journey:

- **Embrace the Unexpected:** Children with Down syndrome often have a unique way of seeing the world. Be open to their perspective and find humor in their innocent observations or unexpected actions.

- **Laugh at Yourself:** Do not be afraid to laugh at yourself! Things might not always go according to plan, and that is okay. A little self-deprecating humor can lighten the mood.

- **Find the Joy in Challenges:** Even challenging situations can hold a humorous nugget. Maybe a meltdown turns into a silly dance party, or a communication breakdown leads to a hilarious misunderstanding.

Fun Activities and Games

Laughter is contagious, so spread the joy! Here are some ideas to incorporate humor into your family time:

- **Playful Games:** Engage in silly games like charades, dress-up, or making funny faces.

- **Watch Funny Movies or Shows:** Cuddle up on the couch and enjoy some lighthearted entertainment together.

- **Read Silly Stories:** Books with playful rhymes, funny characters, or unexpected twists can spark laughter and joy.

- **Tell Jokes (Even Bad Ones!):** Whether it is a classic knock-knock joke or a goofy story you made up, share some laughter together. Do not worry if the jokes are a little corny – the joy of sharing them is what matters most.

Remember

- **Laughter is a Journey, Not a Destination:** Do not force humor. Let it flow naturally from shared experiences and genuine connections.

- **Be Age-Appropriate:** Tailor your humor to your child's age and understanding. Simple jokes and lighthearted silliness work best for younger children, while older children might appreciate more complex humor.

- **Embrace the Absurd:** Sometimes, the funniest moments are the most unexpected. Embrace the absurdity of certain situations and find joy in the laughter it brings.

Beyond the Chapter: A Journey Filled with Joy

This chapter has reminded you of the power of laughter on your journey with Down syndrome. Remember, laughter is a powerful tool that can bring your family closer, create lasting memories, and help you navigate challenges with a lighter heart. So, do not be afraid to embrace the funny, share silly moments, and fill your family circus tent with the joyful sounds of laughter. Laughter truly is the best medicine, and it is a prescription you can use every day!

34. PERSONAL GROWTH AND VALUABLE INSIGHTS

Imagine your child as a wise teacher, offering valuable life lessons. This chapter explores the unique perspective gained from raising a child with Down syndrome. Just like a good teacher imparts knowledge, your child can teach you incredible lessons about patience, love, acceptance, and the true meaning of happiness. By embracing the journey, you will discover personal growth and gain valuable insights that will enrich your life in countless ways.

A Journey of Unexpected Gifts

Raising a child with Down syndrome can be a life-changing experience filled with both challenges and rewards. Here is why this journey offers unexpected gifts:

- **Unconditional Love:** Your child's love is pure and unconditional. They teach you to love without reservation and appreciate the simple joys in life.

- **Strength and Resilience:** Navigating challenges with your child builds your strength, resilience, and problem-solving skills.

- **Patience and Acceptance:** You learn the importance of patience and acceptance, not just for your child, but for everyone in your life.

- **Gratitude and Perspective:** Seeing the world through your child's eyes can shift your perspective and make you appreciate the simple things.

Unforgettable Lessons: Embracing the Journey

Here are some of the most valuable lessons you might learn from raising a child with Down syndrome:

- **The Power of Perseverance:** Your child's determination to overcome challenges inspires you to never give up on your own dreams.

- **The Joy of Small Victories:** You learn to celebrate small victories and appreciate the beauty in everyday moments.

- **The Importance of Advocacy:** You become a fierce advocate for your child and others with Down syndrome, raising awareness and fighting for equality.

- **Living in the Moment:** Your child's focus on the present moment reminds you to slow down, savor experiences, and find joy in the here and now.

Expanding Your Circle and Inspiring Others

The lessons you learn can benefit others as well. Here are ways to share your gifts:

- **Support Groups:** Connect with other parents and share your experiences, offering support and encouragement.

- **Raising Awareness:** Share your story to raise awareness about Down syndrome and break down stereotypes.

- **Spreading Positivity:** Inspire others with your resilience and the joy your child brings to your life.

Remember

- **Every Journey is Unique:** The lessons you learn will be specific to you and your child. Embrace the uniqueness of your journey.

- **Lifelong Learning:** The learning process does not stop. Continue to grow, adapt, and discover new lessons as your child grows and develops.

- **Focus on the Positive:** While challenges are inevitable, focus on the incredible gifts your child offers.

Beyond the Chapter: A Tapestry Woven with Love and Learning

This chapter has highlighted the transformative power of raising a child with Down syndrome. Remember, your child is not just a student; they are a teacher. By embracing the journey and opening your heart to the lessons they offer, you will experience personal growth, gain valuable insights, and weave a beautiful tapestry of love, learning, and joy with your child. The lessons learned on this journey will stay with you forever, enriching your life and inspiring others along the way.

35. LEAVING YOUR MARK

Imagine tossing a pebble into a still pond, sending ripples outward. This chapter explores how you can create a positive impact on the Down Syndrome community. Just like a single pebble can create ripples across the water, your actions, big or small, can make a big difference in the lives of others. By getting involved and using your unique talents, you can contribute to a more inclusive and supportive world for individuals with Down syndrome.

Why Make a Difference?

The Down Syndrome community is strong and vibrant. Here is why getting involved matters:

- **Building a Stronger Network:** Together, you can advocate for change, share resources, and create a more supportive environment for all.

- **Spreading Awareness and Acceptance:** By sharing your story and raising awareness, you can combat stereotypes and promote inclusion.

- **Empowering Others:** Your efforts can inspire others to get involved and contribute to the greater good.

Exploring Ways to Make a Difference

There are many ways to leave your mark, no matter your time or resources. Here are some ideas to get you started:

- **Volunteer:** Donate your time and talents to organizations that support individuals with Down syndrome.

- **Spread Awareness:** Talk to friends, family, and colleagues about Down syndrome. Challenge misconceptions and promote understanding.

- **Fundraise:** Organize or participate in fundraising events to support research, advocacy efforts, or programs for individuals with Down syndrome.

- **Become an Advocate:** Speak up for the rights of individuals with Down syndrome. Contact your local representatives about important legislation.

- **Share Your Story:** Write about your experiences, create a blog, or share your story on social media to raise awareness and inspire others.

- **Embrace Inclusion:** Create opportunities for your child to interact with others outside the Down syndrome community. Promote friendships and acceptance in your everyday life.

Remember

- **Every Contribution Matters:** No act of kindness is too small. Every effort contributes to a more positive future for the Down Syndrome community.

- **Focus on Your Strengths:** What are you passionate about? Use your unique talents and skills to make a difference.

- **Be Patient and Persistent:** Creating change takes time and effort. Stay committed to your cause and inspire others to join you.

Beyond the Chapter: Ripples of Change

This chapter has empowered you to make a positive impact. Remember, you are not alone. Together, you can create a ripple effect of change, building a more inclusive and supportive world for individuals with Down syndrome. By leaving your mark, you will inspire others, empower the community, and pave the way for a brighter future.

Resources

United States:

- **National Down Syndrome Society (NDSS):** https://ndss.org/ - This leading advocacy organization provides resources and support for all aspects of living with Down syndrome.

Canada:

- **Down Syndrome Research Canada (DSRC):** https://cdss.ca/down-syndrome-research/ - DSRC is a national leader in Down syndrome research and advocacy, offering resources for families and professionals.

United Kingdom:

- **Down's Syndrome Association (DSA):** https://www.downs-syndrome.org.uk/ - The DSA is the largest Down syndrome charity in the UK, offering information, support, and resources for families and individuals.

Australia:

- **Down Syndrome Australia (DSA):** https://www.downsyndrome.org.au/ - DSA provides a national voice for people with Down syndrome in Australia, offering resources, support programs, and information.

New Zealand:

- **Down Syndrome Association of New Zealand (DSANZ):** https://nzdsa.org.nz/ - DSANZ offers support, information, and advocacy services for families and individuals with Down syndrome in New Zealand.

South Africa:

- **Down Syndrome South Africa (DSSA):** https://www.downsyndrome.org.za/ - DSSA is a national organization providing support, resources, and advocacy for individuals with Down syndrome and their families in South Africa.

India:

- **Down Syndrome Federation of India (DSFI):** https://downsyndrome.in/ - DSFI is a national advocacy group working to improve the lives of people with Down syndrome in India. They offer resources, information, and programs for families and professionals.

CAN YOU HELP OTHERS FIND THIS BOOK BY WRITING A REVIEW?

Thank you for reading the book. As a retired physician with a fresh viewpoint, I am dedicating my time to creating this informative series out of a desire to empower others through credible information. This series is my way of continuing to serve others, not for profit, but out of a deep love and passion for sharing knowledge to benefit those who are perplexed by the overwhelming information overload in the digital world. Therefore, I have created this series of patient information books as a one-stop information haven, painstakingly built to save you valuable time. Your honest review on Amazon, accessible through the QR code below, will be a guiding light for others seeking clarity. Let us empower each other, one informed reader at a time! Kindly write a review about this book!

ABOUT THE AUTHOR

Dr. A. Mitra is a retired medical doctor who has worked in the field of General Practice in Family Medicine in India and Australia for over 30 years. He completed his graduate education in India and then did further studies in Australia and UK. Currently he lives a private modest life and pursues his interests in reading and writing on various topics.